BODYWEIGHT TRAINING OVER 40

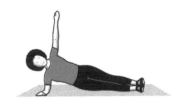

BODYWEIGHT
TRAINING
OVER 40

Build Strength, Balance,
and Flexibility with Zero Equipment

Mel McGuire

Illustrations by Mat Edwards

ROCKRIDGE
PRESS

Interior and Cover Designer: Amanda Kirk
Art Producer: Samantha Ulban
Editor: Eun H. Jeong
Production Editor: Jenna Dutton
Production Manager: David Zapanta

Illustrations © 2022 Mat Edwards. Author photo courtesy of Stephen Emerick.

Paperback ISBN: 978-1-63878-886-7
eBook ISBN: 978-1-63878-504-0
R0

For my son, Phillip, who is still working on lifting
his head during "tummy time," and my stepdaughter,
Emily, who just began her second decade on a pair
of very long legs. I hope I can pass on to both of you my
love of fitness so that you have strong and active
bodies to take you into the twenty-second century.

CONTENTS

INTRODUCTION

When I was growing up, I observed that my family was fairly sedentary. The grown-ups seemed to sit all day: in cars, at desks, at dinner tables, and then watching TV at night. From my perspective, their bodies didn't seem to do much for them. My parents didn't engage in physical activities with me, and I grew up feeling insecure about my ability to participate in them. I also took on the viewpoint that growing older meant moving less.

When I was sixteen years old, my family took a trip to California and stopped for a day to visit Hearst Castle in San Simeon. I had done some research and was so excited to explore the palatial estate. Unfortunately, my father's health had deteriorated so much from complications of diabetes that he could no longer climb stairs. We were forced to take the short and limited tour of the castle that showcased only the first floor. My father and I were both crushed to miss the opportunity to see every inch of this epic landmark. I realized that one's health affects not only their own life but the lives of those around them as well. It was on this day that I dedicated myself to fitness.

I started working out in my teens and turned to fitness as a career in my twenties. I've now been a personal trainer and group exercise instructor for twenty years. I'm certified to work with people who have various medical conditions, and I collaborate with their medical teams to create programs complementing their treatment plans. I also work with clients of all ages, including many over the age of forty. I remind them that aging doesn't mean our health has to decline.

Regardless of the reason you picked up this book and no matter where you are now in your fitness journey, thank you for allowing me to guide you on your path to being your best self. Fitness is always a personal journey that will be unique and special to you. My goal for you with this book is to help you create a strong physical foundation and a bodyweight fitness program that works for you so you can move better, more often, and with strength and ease for many years to come. I hope that you will be able to explore every castle that comes your way, whether you are forty-five, sixty-five, eighty-five, or one hundred and five.

HOW TO USE THIS BOOK

It's important to start at the beginning and read the first three chapters in part 1. Chapter 1 will allow you to properly assess yourself as you start out and make you aware of all the things to consider about your body that may affect how you respond to the exercises in this book. In chapter 2, we'll cover components of lasting change to strength, flexibility, balance, and endurance, such as nutrition and good exercise habits. In chapter 3, you'll find a variety of stretches and bodyweight exercises that cover the whole body. Each exercise includes illustrations, step-by-step instructions, and details on where to focus your attention, what you will feel, and what to avoid. Modifications and tips are also offered on many exercises. These explain how to make an activity easier or more challenging, as well as how to move your body in a way that's effective and prevents injury.

In part 2, you'll find twelve weeks of bodyweight workouts. The workouts will progress in skill and intensity as you get stronger and fitter, beginning with three weeks of beginner programs, then intermediate, advanced, and, finally, expert.

Even if you consider yourself an expert or advanced in your fitness level, I still recommend starting from the beginner programs in chapter 4 and following the workouts in order. This way, you'll build a solid foundation for specific muscles to thrive as the intensity increases.

The end of each level's chapter offers opportunity for self-reflection and note-taking. Sometimes it's tempting to just plow ahead and "level up"—however, there may also be reasons to stay where you are and spend more time with the basics. Remember that it isn't just about getting stronger; it's about feeling good in your body, too. So many factors can affect a workout, such as stress, sleep, nutrition, injury, and other medical issues, and everyone's body responds differently.

Repetition and consistency often get the best results, so please don't be discouraged if you have to use an easier modification. As long as you stick with the program, you will see progress. For muscular balance, it's important to follow the exercises prescribed in each week's sequence to get a total body workout and not just choose the ones that feel personally satisfying. We all have strengths, weaknesses, and personal preferences, but it's just as important (maybe even more important) to work on the exercises that challenge us the most. However, it's also important to pay attention to the body's signals to make sure we are working out safely. Dizziness, inability to catch your breath, and chest pain while you are working out are always reasons to contact a doctor immediately.

One of the best parts of this book is that no equipment is needed for the exercises. You can really do this anywhere. Granted, some of the exercises may include recommendations to use a chair, step, wall, or other pieces of available furniture to reduce the angle of resistance or help with balance or support. You also might want to have padding on the floor for some exercises—this can just be a mat, carpet, or towel. But forget the home gym equipment. You've got all you need!

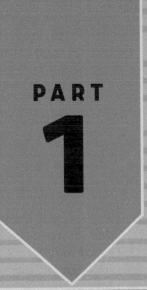

PART 1

Foundation for Success

EXERCISE IS A CRITICAL COMPONENT OF A well-rounded approach to improving your health. In part 1, we'll go over the importance of building muscle for strength, mobility, and overall health. You'll read about how exercise can help you head off some common health issues as you age and how bodyweight training can be especially beneficial for your overall health. There will also be guidance on building a fitness program that is right for you, incorporating good nutrition, activity, and adequate rest into your life. You will also find detailed instructions for numerous bodyweight exercises that work out the whole body as well as tips that will help you modify the movement for your comfort.

STRONGER FOR LONGER

In this chapter, we'll talk about the importance of strong muscles for our health, especially as we age. We'll discuss the various effects that aging can have on the body, as well as some of the more common health issues for people over forty. We will also explore how exercise can help us build muscle and head off health issues. You'll then determine your personal readiness for bringing a bodyweight training program into your life so you can build one that's right for you.

MORE THAN JUST MUSCLE

Muscles do more than just help us move our body. They are critical to our overall health, contributing to strength, endurance, stamina, balance, flexibility, and mobility, as well as helping manage our metabolism. Muscle also plays a role in joint integrity and keeping pain out of our joints. Unfortunately, starting in our thirties, our body starts to naturally lose a little bit of muscle due to a biological process called **sarcopenia**. As the muscle loss progresses, our body can feel weaker and is more prone to pain and injury. The decline of muscle mass also has negative effects on balance, flexibility, and posture. Having less **lean body mass** also slows down our metabolism, making it harder to maintain a healthy weight, so much so that this small yearly muscle loss is often accompanied by a small yearly weight gain.

But there is good news! Muscle loss can be reversed. Muscles can regenerate and grow to new, greater capacities at any age when challenged with regular fitness endeavors, such as bodyweight training. Bodyweight training uses the resistance of the body and gravity to put stress on the muscles in a way that stimulates muscle growth. The muscles' ability to regenerate means it's never too late to start building muscle. As you build your muscles with exercise, you'll also notice improvements in your endurance, stamina, metabolism, balance, flexibility, and posture, and your joints will be able to function appropriately and serve you a whole lot longer.

Connections between Muscles, Hormones, and Metabolism

Hormones play a key role in all physiological processes, including how the aging process affects muscles and metabolism. As we age, the hormones that help build muscle—like testosterone, estrogen, and the growth hormone—decrease, while thyroid hormones and glucocorticoids—which can slow metabolism—increase. This imbalance in hormone production has an inflammatory effect on the body. Inflammation causes issues like soreness, fatigue, and even bloating, which lend themselves to a sedentary lifestyle, consequently allowing the muscle loss of sarcopenia to have a greater effect. Without active muscle building, weakness and risk of injury and pain increase.

Regular physical activity builds muscle, but this activity also helps release hormones that produce an anti-inflammatory response in the body. Additionally, it decreases the production of the stress hormone cortisol, improving your overall mood and sense of well-being. As your body becomes more efficient at producing a better hormonal balance through exercise, your metabolism will become more efficient as well, helping you maintain a healthy weight.

Strength, Balance, and Mobility

In addition to its positive effects on regulating hormones and metabolism, working out is also critical for maintaining strength, balance, and mobility.

Your body's mobility is directly related to the strength and flexibility of your muscles, which in turn protect your aging joints. Muscles move your joints, and this is one of the reasons it's important to build muscle strength and mass to maintain mobility as you age. Muscles also help absorb the force on your joints as you move, and without enough muscle, the joints will bear more of the impact, leading to pain and excess wear and tear. Bodyweight training exercises can help build muscles and keep them strong around your joints to maintain mobility. The great thing about bodyweight training to keep your joints healthy is that by using your own body, you are working only within your own range of motion and physical control. It eliminates some of the risk that comes with adding external forces, like barbells, that can overload the skeletal system.

Strong muscles, especially in the back and core, also help maintain good posture, which is essential for keeping balance and decreasing the risk of falling. Regularly practicing bodyweight balance exercises with uneven weight shifts and single-leg stances can help improve balance.

HEADING OFF HEALTH ISSUES

There are many types of exercises, such as **weight training**, **resistance training**, and **cardiovascular training**. You can even combine them to cater to your specific goals and needs. We've touched on how exercise improves numerous areas of our health, including strength, mobility, balance, mental well-being, and metabolism. Another advantage of exercise is its preventive impact on common health issues, such as **hypertension**, **diabetes**, heart health, bone density, and brain health. These health issues can be a concern at any age, but they become much more prevalent in people over forty, because age increases our risk factors for each one.

Bodyweight training can be your secret weapon against many of these chronic medical conditions. A bodyweight training program is easily tailored to whatever demands your body faces on a regular basis. By engaging in simple movements you can do without any equipment, you'll build physical power. Bodyweight training is unique in that with it, no muscle can ever truly be isolated, and so every movement, no matter how small, sets your total body up to receive all the benefits of the exercise. With additional muscles working to stabilize your body as others control your movements, your metabolism will be fired up while you perform almost any bodyweight exercise. As noted earlier, you can also use bodyweight exercises to improve your cardiovascular performance by incorporating them into a **circuit training** program. In a circuit training program, you perform exercises back-to-back with short rest periods, keeping your heart rate up. By making time for a regular routine, you'll be taking significant positive steps toward a healthier, happier future.

Hypertension

Bodyweight training to improve muscle mass and **cardiovascular** endurance has a direct and positive effect on hypertension, or high blood pressure. Simply put, exercise makes your heart stronger, which helps it work more efficiently to move blood through your arteries with ease. You don't need to run a marathon to achieve this! Regular, low- to moderate-intensity cardio exercise has been proven to lower blood pressure and control hypertension. When performed consistently, a regular routine of simple cardio exercises such as brisk walking and bodyweight circuit training can help bring hypertension under control after just a few months. Exercise also helps with weight management and stress reduction, both of which have a positive effect on blood pressure. This said, it's important to remember that the positive effects that exercise has on blood pressure last only as long as regular exercise is maintained.

Diabetes

For the purposes of this book, when diabetes is referenced, we will be talking about type 2.

Type 2 diabetes is a disease in which blood sugar levels can become chronically too high. Insulin is a hormone that helps the body process sugar. With diabetes, the body either doesn't produce enough insulin to turn blood sugar (**glucose**) into energy or the cells stop responding to insulin. Blood glucose is our primary source of energy, so not being able to process it properly results in various physical complications. High body fat and obesity can lead to diabetes. It's also a progressive disease—it gets worse over time.

If the condition is not overly advanced, there are lots of measures you can take to lower your blood sugar levels. Low- to moderate-level cardio exercise can reduce blood sugar, and adjusting your diet can have a great impact as well. Even if you are genetically predisposed to diabetes, a lifestyle of regular exercise and good nutrition greatly improves your chance of avoiding this difficult disease.

Heart Health

Along with hypertension and diabetes, the risk for heart disease, stroke, and other vascular conditions increases with age. Being overweight also puts undue stress on the heart. However, a combination of exercise and good nutrition can lower the risks and help maintain a healthy weight. As mentioned above, simple cardio exercise like bodyweight circuit training can help lower hypertension, as well as strengthen the heart. After all, the heart is just another muscle!

One way to measure if you have a healthy heart is finding out your resting heart rate. In most cases, the lower your resting heart rate, the greater your cardiovascular fitness. Average healthy heart rates are between sixty and eighty beats per minute, but generally speaking, the lower the better. Just beginning an exercise program can contribute to a lower resting heart rate, and as you get more physically fit, it will continue to go down. A lower resting pulse translates to less internal effort to get through the physical demands of life.

Bone Density

Bone is a regenerating compound in the body, and it's constantly breaking down and regrowing throughout our life. Like muscle mass loss, bone density loss is a natural part of the aging process. Without prevention, the risk increases for developing **osteoporosis**, a condition in which the body isn't creating enough new bone to replace the loss of the old bone. With osteoporosis, the bones become brittle and weak, putting us at an increased risk of falls and fractures.

Diet, exercise, supplements, and other healthy lifestyle habits can prevent more bone loss from occurring and even stimulate new bone growth.

Bodyweight training can foster bone growth in the same way it does for muscle growth. By putting load, or stress, on our skeleton, we stimulate the healthy breakdown and rebuilding of strong bones. The muscles pulling on the bones also stimulates them to bulk up.

Brain Health

Perhaps the most important organ to keep healthy as we age? Our brain! Like the other areas of our health, such as heart and bone health, exercise can have a positive impact on the brain. First, all the positive effects of exercise on the heart also impact the brain. As more blood is pumped throughout the body, the brain gets more oxygen. Second, the hormones released to the brain during exercise stimulate new brain-cell growth and even serve as an antidepressant, reducing stress hormones. Exercise is recommended to help stave off depression, increase focus, and improve memory.

Research has also shown that physical fitness can protect against cognitive decline. In a forty-four-year Swedish study, researchers found that women who scored high on a fitness test in midlife were nearly 90 percent less likely to develop dementia than those who weren't as fit, and the fittest women who developed dementia did not do so until ten years later than their less-fit counterparts.

FITNESS TEST

Are you ready? Let's take a deeper look at where your health is today. By taking this short test, you'll discover more personal information on the best and safest way to approach your bodyweight training program.

Answer yes or no to the following questions.

1. Do I have heart disease, hypertension, or diabetes?

2. Do I have any medical condition that could worsen with exercise?

3. Am I on any medications that might impact how my body responds to exercise?

4. Has it been more than five years since I've seen a doctor for a physical?

5. Have I had a recent injury that has not completely healed or that I have not seen a physical therapist about? Or an injury that is still causing me pain?

6. Am I able to safely get up and down off the floor?

7. Do I have a balance issue or **neurological** condition that puts me at a greater risk of falling?

8. Am I over the age of sixty-five and never exercised before?

If you answered yes or were unsure for any of the first five questions, it's a good idea to speak with your health provider before starting an exercise program. Prepare some specific questions about what you might need to focus on or avoid during your workouts. Are there exercises you should specifically avoid in light of a previous injury? Are there limitations to the suggested intensity of your workout? If you are on any medications, ask your health provider or pharmacist about their potential side effects.

If you answered no or were unsure for question 6 and yes or were unsure for question 7, bodyweight training may either not be the best fit for you or not a journey to embark on unsupervised. A better option might be to consult a personal trainer who can design a safe, effective way for you to work out. If you answered yes to question 8, you also might want to consider consulting with a personal trainer for a few guided sessions to learn more about how your body moves and responds to exercise.

There is no single fitness program in the world that is right for everyone. Everybody deserves individual respect and attention when it comes to exercise. Some of us can do this for ourselves, but there is also great value in consulting with a fitness expert to help along the way. If you are a true beginner and have never attempted a squat or plank before, I highly recommend working with a personal trainer a few times before starting your fitness program. The increased confidence, technique, and body awareness you're sure to gain will help ensure success on your journey.

GET PUMPED: GOAL WORKSHEET

Are you excited to get started and experience all the benefits of bodyweight training? Before you start, take a few minutes to reflect on your motivations and goals to help you solidify the commitment to your physical health.

1. Are there places you want to travel and people you want to have adventures with as you age?

2. Can you picture yourself playing sports and enjoying the outdoors with your children, grandchildren, or other kids in your life?

3. Do you want to avoid preventable obstacles to good health?

4. Have you watched a loved one suffer as the result of an unhealthy or inactive lifestyle?

5. Can you remember a time when your body moved with strength and ease?

6. How do you want to feel about yourself and your overall well-being?

7. How much time can you set aside for your health each day?

8. What activities are you interested in that may help you maintain good health?

9. How much improvement in strength and mobility do you want to see in yourself in a month's time? In six months? In a year?

10. Who do I want to share my fitness goals with? Who can I ask for support?

Moving your body with strength and ease doesn't have to be a distant memory just because of age. You've read how being mobile, fit, and healthy as you age can benefit you as well as your loved ones. So before you move on to chapter 2, I invite you to dedicate your fitness program not just to yourself but also to someone you love—someone who will be happy watching you progress and proud of you on your journey.

BUILDING WORKOUTS AND BUILDING MUSCLE

All this talk about exercise! But guess what? Health, longevity, and vitality can't be achieved by exercise alone. In this chapter, we'll explore good nutrition, different exercise methodologies, and rest and recovery tips to help you develop a holistic, well-rounded approach to your health.

We'll also look at some age-specific considerations you should make for building an exercise program that is right for you. All the effort that goes into in a new bodyweight training program will be most effective when it's supported by good nutrition, a complementary movement plan, and a smart strategy for rest and recovery. If your workout program is the star of the show, this chapter will help you develop your supporting players so your lead actor can do their best work.

NUTRITION

As we discussed in chapter 1, sarcopenia and muscle loss are a large part of aging that we can combat with proper diet and exercise. Muscles are best built with a well-rounded, nutrient-dense diet. A food that is nutrient-dense carries a higher load of nutrients, which is beneficial to muscle building and supports bodily functions much more than a food that is just high in calories, or energy. For example, a 100-calorie apple is packed with fiber, vitamin C, and other anti-oxidants, but a 100-calorie serving of jelly beans is full of sugar and chemicals that your body can't use.

Consuming higher-quality food converts to higher-quality building blocks for your body to use for muscle growth and sustenance. There are different approaches to determining which foods are nutrient-dense, but for an easy guideline, avoid heavily processed foods as much as possible and make sure you're getting lots of fresh, whole foods in their natural state. For example, a whole potato nutritionally trumps a bag of potato chips. To learn more about this, let's first walk through the three main nutrients, or **macronutrients**, in a healthy diet: **protein**, carbs, and fat.

Protein

Protein is a macronutrient that's essential primarily for building muscle in the body; however, it also helps build bone tissue, brain tissue, and other vital organs. Good sources of dietary protein include meat, fish, eggs, dairy, beans, nuts, tofu, quinoa, lentils, and certain vegetables. The recommended daily amount of dietary protein is about 15 percent of total calorie intake; however, new research shows that older adults may benefit from protein intake as high as 35 percent.

Carbs

Carbohydrates are another one of the three main macronutrients found in food. Carbohydrates break down to glucose in the body, serving as your body's main source of energy. They make up 45 to 60 percent of total caloric intake in a healthy diet. Carbohydrates have gotten a bad reputation because they are broken down into sugar, and if not used quickly for energy, the excess is stored as fat. Not all foods with carbohydrates are created equal, however, so it's important to choose the right carbs to fuel your muscles. The best source of carbs for this are foods containing some dietary fiber and **micronutrients**, which are vitamins and minerals needed in smaller amounts that contribute to all essential bodily functions.

Grains, potatoes, fruits, vegetables, rice, and bread are a few examples of healthy sources of carbohydrates. Those that are also high in sugar, such as fruit, can be great for a preworkout energy boost, because the body doesn't have to work hard to break them down and can use the sugar immediately. More fiber-rich foods, like brown rice or starchy vegetables, can be more effective after a workout to help replenish your muscles.

Fat

Twenty percent of a healthy diet should ideally come from fat. Proper fat intake helps the body form healthy cell membranes, aids in brain and nervous system function, and regulates hormone production. Fat also helps you feel full after a meal. As with carbohydrates, you'll want to carefully choose the foods you use to meet your daily fat intake requirements.

Some fats are better than others. It's most important to consume essential fats (polyunsaturated and monounsaturated), which can be found in foods such as avocados; olives; peanuts; and soy, safflower, and sunflower oils. Some of your essential fats should come from omega-3 fatty acids, which have many nutritional benefits, especially for heart health. These beneficial omega fats can be found in most fatty fish like salmon, sardines, and mackerel, as well as chia seeds, flaxseed, and walnuts. You can also find healthy saturated fat in animal fat, dairy, and coconut oil. Try to avoid trans fats and fats found in prepackaged snack foods and heavily fried food.

Preworkout

You can maximize your workout performance and properly fuel your muscles by eating a complete meal two to three hours prior. But in the real world, perfect timing isn't always possible. For optimal muscle building in a bodyweight training program, it's best to have something in your stomach to burn, so even if you can't consume a complete meal two to three hours before your workout, you'll have similar success with a light meal an hour before. Choose foods that are easy to digest to avoid an upset stomach once you start your workout (see the Light Meal Suggestions on this page).

If you're eating less than 45 minutes before your workout, opt for a fast-burning snack for fuel, and then focus on getting your complete nutrition postworkout. Everyone's body responds to food differently, so you may have to experiment with some different meal choices to find out what works best for you (see the Snack Suggestions on page 14).

LIGHT MEAL SUGGESTIONS (1 HOUR BEFORE WORKOUT)

» 2 hard-boiled eggs and 1 slice of whole-grain toast

» 1 slice of whole-grain toast with ½ avocado and 1 ounce of smoked salmon

» Grilled chicken breast, 1 cup of steamed broccoli, and ½ cup of cooked wild rice

» Scrambled eggs, steamed spinach, and ½ baked sweet potato

» 2 chicken sausages and ½ cup of cooked vegetable quinoa

» 1 cup of oatmeal with walnuts, chia seeds, and strawberries

» Collagen protein smoothie with banana, almond butter, and flaxseed oil

» ¾ cup of granola with 1 cup of whole milk

» Grilled portobello mushroom with arugula salad, olive oil, and sprinkled Parmesan cheese

» 1 cup of tuna salad with olive oil mayo on a whole-grain English muffin

SNACK SUGGESTIONS (LESS THAN 45 MINUTES BEFORE WORKOUT)

» Apple with 1 tablespoon of almond butter

» Banana

» 1 cup of yogurt with ¼ cup of blueberries or raspberries

» Baby carrots with ¼ cup of hummus

» Sliced bell pepper with ½ avocado

Postworkout

Ideally, postworkout nutrition should be focused on healing muscles and replenishing energy stores. If you've been regularly eating all day prior to your workout, it's not necessary to eat immediately after, but generally you'll want to eat within an hour of completing your workout.

   If you don't have time for a full meal, snacks can be eaten anytime between 15 minutes and 1 hour after your workout to sustain you until your next meal. Check out the following light meals and snacks, perfect for after a workout.

LIGHT MEALS (WITHIN 1 HOUR AFTER WORKOUT)

» Whole-grain veggie wrap with shrimp or chicken

» Mixed green salad with grilled chicken, walnuts, balsamic vinaigrette, and feta cheese

» 4 ounces of lean steak with grilled asparagus and brown rice

» Turkey breast, ½ baked potato, and steamed asparagus

» Cod fillet, sautéed spinach, and ½ cup of couscous

» ¼ pound of lean hamburger over kale salad and ½ sweet potato

» Roasted chicken breast and steamed broccoli

» 4 to 6 ounces of salmon, wild rice, and stir-fried vegetables

» Vegetable quiche and baby greens

» Bacon, lettuce, sliced turkey, avocado, and tomato sandwich on seeded whole-grain bread

SNACKS (15 MINUTES TO 1 HOUR AFTER WORKOUT)

» 2 mozzarella string cheese sticks and an apple

» ¼ cup of raw almonds and 2 small dark chocolate squares

» ¼ cup of guacamole with baked tortilla chips

» Sugar snap peas with ¼ cup of hummus

» ½ cup of olives and multigrain baked crackers

Hydration

Proper hydration supports all systems in the body to do their best work during both physical and mental performance and recovery. Even on days when you don't work out, it's important to properly hydrate your body by drinking at least eight glasses of water. On days when you do work out, sweat a lot, or consume caffeine or alcohol, your water needs will increase. Water lost in sweat also needs to be replaced on top of your daily requirements. Thirst isn't always a good indicator of dehydration, so don't wait until you're thirsty to get a drink. And for best results, rather than chugging your water all at once, try to consume small amounts of water throughout the day.

Supplements

In addition to the three macronutrients (protein, carbohydrates, and fat), there are also twenty-six essential micronutrients in the form of vitamins and minerals that the body requires for optimal vitality and nutritional balance. Even with a regular diet of healthy meals, it can be hard to meet all of your micronutrient needs, and some supplementation might be needed. Following are a few supplements to consider asking your health provider about adding to your daily intake. This way, you can feel your best and get the most out of your bodyweight training program. It's also a good idea to research different brands of supplements, because the market is flooded with many brands that are not all high quality.

» **Calcium and magnesium**—Especially as we age, calcium supplementation can become essential to prevent osteoporosis and bone degeneration. Calcium needs magnesium to deliver it to the right parts of the body, so these supplements should be taken together.

» **Vitamin D**—Vitamin D helps the body absorb calcium and is essential for bone health. It also supports the immune system, helps with muscular and brain function, and has anti-inflammatory properties. Your body can make vitamin D when it absorbs direct sunlight, but it's hard to get enough dietary vitamin D without supplementation.

» **Omega-3 fatty acids**—Omega-3 fatty acids may help lower the risk of heart disease, depression, arthritis, and stroke. See page 12 for some sources of omega-3s. They can be hard to get in your diet without supplementation, so if this is an issue for you, a fish oil or flaxseed oil supplement can help.

» **Vitamin B**—Vitamin B has a positive impact on brain function and metabolism and is important for creating new red blood cells to deliver oxygen to muscles. Your immune system may also benefit from a vitamin B supplement. There are different B vitamins, including B_{12} and B_6, that can be gotten through diet. Talk to your doctor about your vitamin B levels and to find out if supplementation might benefit your health.

» **Collagen**—Collagen is the main structural protein found in skin and connective body tissues. The benefits of collagen supplementation include supporting bone and joint health, strengthening nails and hair, promoting skin elasticity, and improving immune function. Collagen is available in pill form but is also sold in protein powders that can be mixed into smoothies or other foods.

AGE-SPECIFIC CONSIDERATIONS

A bodyweight training program is one of the most effective and safest ways to maintain fitness over the age of forty. Negative effects of aging start to appear incrementally every year after age thirty, especially for people who lead a more sedentary lifestyle. But even in an active person, there are changes in the body that hormonally and structurally come into play over time. As you age, your needs and abilities will change. I've broken down these changes decade by decade to provide general guidance on where to focus your workout depending on your age, but everyone will experience these changes differently. Use the following information to help you recognize changes as you experience them, and adapt your fitness program accordingly.

Forties

In your forties, you may notice your metabolism is slowing down. This is due to hormonal changes in your body. You may also find that physical exertion takes a greater toll on you than it did in your twenties and thirties. For a proper recovery, a vigorous workout will require more rest than it did in your twenties and thirties. If you exert yourself in the same way you did in your twenties and thirties during your workout, you may be prone to injury due to overuse or improper support.

In your forties, you'll benefit most from high-intensity, short workouts that fire up your metabolism and stimulate muscle growth but don't deplete all your energy. Your body will also benefit from longer warm-ups before an intense workout and more time focusing on flexibility to avoid injury. Adjustment can feel awkward at first and take some getting used to, but the foundation you build to pay attention to your body's changing needs and abilities will set your body up to feel good in the years to come.

Fifties

In your fifties, it's more important than ever to stay active. Heart health is a priority, as this is the decade that risk for stroke and heart disease increases. You can improve your cardiovascular fitness with bodyweight circuit training workouts, jogging, cycling, hiking, and even brisk walking. The beginnings of arthritis can arise in your fifties, so you'll want to protect your joints with exercises that work you through a full range of motion at every joint. Working through the full range of motion prevents tightening and shortening of major muscle groups. Strong muscles will also help absorb the impact on your joints from higher-intensity activities, making strength training an excellent investment.

Many women end **perimenopause** and reach menopause in their fifties, which could mean they now have more energy than they did in their forties. Postmenopausal women will need to focus more on bone health as the risk of osteoporosis increases. Engaging in weight-bearing activities will stimulate bone growth and is a key component of an effective circuit training program.

Sixties

Osteoarthritis and osteoporosis become more prevalent in the sixties, so you'll want to keep your joints mobile and lubricated and your bones strong. Your immune system also might become weaker, so staying hydrated, eating nutritious foods rich in antioxidants, and getting ample rest are all essential for overall health. The combination of a weakened immune system and weakened joints makes recovery from illness and injury a longer process. Be patient with yourself—you can absolutely build strength and improve flexibility at this age. If you have started to feel some aging effects on your joints, choose lower-impact cardio activities than you did before.

Also, be sure to focus on weight-bearing exercises for skeletal health. Because of gravity's lifelong effect on the spine, you may lose some height in your sixties, but working on exercises that target postural muscles (those that support your shoulders, back, torso, and butt) will help you maintain good body alignment.

Seventies and Beyond

It's especially important in your seventies and beyond to stay active to preserve muscles, build confidence, promote physical and mental well-being, and maintain independence. Continue doing the things you love, but as at any age, train and rest at a pace that is right for you and your specific needs.

Flexibility and balance training are both critical for daily activities such as navigating stairs and getting up from chairs. They will help prevent falls and other injuries that can involve a long recovery time. Staying active can also help alleviate symptoms of osteoarthritis and other physical ailments. Long warm-ups that lead into movement will help with joint aches; cooldowns that focus on flexibility will have the greatest impact on keeping your body in balance.

All the benefits of exercise in earlier decades still apply; for example, you can absolutely build muscle and improve mobility, flexibility, and heart health, to name just a few. Just give yourself the grace and support to build a fitness routine that honors your specific needs and abilities. Consulting a trainer and/or doctor can be especially beneficial in helping you establish a fitness program that is right for you.

EXERCISE MODALITIES

To get the most from your bodyweight training program, it helps to understand some of the circuit training modalities we'll be applying to your workouts. Learning these different training approaches and their benefits will enhance your motivation to stick with the program.

Peripheral Heart Action Training

Peripheral heart action (PHA) training is a technique applied to circuit training workouts to improve a person's aerobic capacity. Although conceived in the 1940s, PHA training has recently been studied as an alternative to the popular high-intensity interval training (HIIT) training. The desired benefits of HIIT training are to improve athletic performance and maximize calorie burning by firing up metabolism. In a HIIT workout, you achieve these results by giving maximum effort for short periods of time with little rest in between.

Although it is effective, HIIT can overstress the body, and too many or too intense HIIT sessions can backfire and lead to overtraining. When the muscles and nervous system are overtrained, the entire body can experience a systemic burnout, leaving you with low energy, pain, and fatigue. In addition, you just might find the intensity of HIIT workouts unsustainable.

The benefits of PHA training are similar to the metabolic stimulation achieved through an HIIT workout, but the intensity is lower, so there are fewer risks of injury. A typical PHA workout involves alternating from an upper-body exercise to a lower-body exercise with very little rest time until you complete the circuit. This increases blood flow to the extremities and has a positive effect on cardiovascular fitness. Because of the added blood circulation, when applied to your bodyweight training program, PHA will burn more calories and deliver other metabolic and aerobic benefits.

Push/Pull Training

Push/pull training is a strength-training technique that keeps the body in balance and involves working opposing muscle groups to their greatest potential. In bodyweight and circuit training, for every pushing exercise you do, you follow it with a pulling exercise. Most pushing exercises train the muscles on the front of the body. For example, a push-up works your chest, shoulders, and abdominal muscles. When you do the alternative pulling movement, such as a body row, you're working the lats, rhomboids, and posterior deltoids—all muscles on the back of the body. Alternating between pushing and pulling movements helps your posture and protects your joints from overuse injuries.

Like PHA training, this type of training stimulates blood flow—it does so by working opposing movements in the same workout, but the strength and stretch benefits of push/pull training are also important and help in optimal muscle recovery. When pushing, you are contracting the push muscles but stretching the pull muscles, and vice versa. So, when alternating between the two, you will additionally stimulate your stretch reflex and improve range of motion in the stretching muscles.

Eccentric Training

In eccentric training, the focus is on slowing down the body's movement against gravity. This strength-training method can be applied to your bodyweight workouts to add intensity and create more time under tension in your muscles for greater strength gains. For example, while performing a bodyweight squat, you would concentrate on descending as slowly as you can control to the bottom of the movement and then lift yourself up at a normal pace.

Eccentric training can help you focus on the quality of the exercise you are performing. When you slow down, you can use the time to really feel the muscle you are working. This heightened awareness of muscle use while going at a slower pace can help you get the most out of your bodyweight workout.

REST AND RECOVERY

Bodyweight training workouts increase strength and flexibility in your body, but every good workout plan needs to be balanced with a good recovery strategy. After you tax your muscles in a bodyweight workout, they need ample time to rest. In fact, it's during rest that muscles do the important business of rebuilding and getting stronger. Though its effects are positive, exercise is a stressor on the body, and if the demands of everyday life are also putting stress on you, the body and mind can get overloaded. When a muscle is too overloaded or fatigued to do its job properly, the body makes compensations, which can lead to injury.

To prevent overload, you can integrate complementary movement into your schedule to strengthen surrounding structures in the body or challenge other parts that may be not getting used during our regular workouts. Doing this also allows you to continue building flexibility, endurance, and stamina even on days off, as well as mixes things up by integrating other enjoyable activities. We'll talk more about this in the next section.

Hydration, sleep, and nutrition also play big roles in the body's ability to bounce back in time for the next workout or physical challenge. As we've discussed, your need for rest and recovery will change as you age, so it's important to listen to your body and integrate rest and recovery into your fitness routine in order to maintain and continue a healthy, active lifestyle.

Complementary Movement

We just talked about incorporating "complementary movement" into your weekly schedule to get the most out of a bodyweight training program and make the fitness routine more fun. Some of the following options can be done on active rest days, and some will be workouts on their own.

» **Cardiovascular training**—Aerobics, jogging, cycling, hiking, and brisk walking are all great ways to strengthen your heart and help with your stamina and endurance. Low-impact cardio can be done on your active rest days; more vigorous cardio can serve as a workout on its own. Try to get at least 30 minutes of focused cardiovascular training two to three times a week in addition to your bodyweight training.

» **Yoga/Tai Chi/Pilates**—These exercise modalities improve flexibility and incorporate the mind-body connection, breathing techniques, and deep core activation. Additionally, they will help you restore posture, flexibility, and balance, as well as relieve mental stress. Restorative yoga and meditation are great for active rest days. The intensity of regular yoga and Pilates can vary greatly, so consider this when planning your workouts. I recommend 45 minutes to an hour twice a week.

» **Myofascial release/massage**—Myofascial release with a self-massage tool or foam roller can help restore balance to fascia, or connective tissues, of muscles after a hard workout. This can be especially helpful if you have a recurring injury or a known muscular imbalance. Putting massage pressure on an affected muscle can relieve tightness and stimulate blood flow to that area. This can be useful to do right before a workout or in an isolated massage session. See the resources section (page 164) for more information on this subject.

» **Sports and recreation**—Exercise can and should be fun! Making time for playing a sport or athletic pastime that you love or enjoy can help you stay in shape and keep you motivated to continue your strength training. Tennis, golf, swimming, and other social sports are also great ways to get outside in the fresh air, soak up some vitamin D, and connect with friends and others who value remaining active as much as you do. These activities are great for active rest days.

Rest

Bodyweight training isn't meant to be an everyday routine. Muscles need recovery time after a strength-training workout, so give yourself one or two days of rest between your bodyweight training sessions. But unless you're sick or overworked, "rest" doesn't have to mean sitting around all day! Active rest days can be exceptionally healing, and complementary movement like cardiovascular exercise or a yoga class can be done in between your bodyweight workouts. If you're taking a rest day, you can still enjoy low-impact movement like walking and stretching. Light movement will help your cells regenerate faster and can alleviate soreness from previous workouts faster than if you're sedentary.

Sleep

During deep sleep, the pituitary gland releases a growth hormone essential for tissue growth and muscle repair. If you don't get enough sleep, the production of growth hormone is impaired, which can lead to increased muscle loss. Between six and a half and nine hours of sleep is recommended for optimal muscle recovery. Adequate sleep also improves cognitive function, metabolism, and skin repair, and refreshes your immune system, keeping you protected from illness. Insomnia is common in older adults, so try to create sleep conditions that support a good night's sleep. This can include avoiding caffeine and alcohol late in the day, keeping a screen-free and blue-light-free sleep zone, and sleeping in a comfortable bed. See the resources section (page 164) for some helpful apps to promote sleep.

Self-Evaluation

Starting a fitness program and building muscle in your body can be fatiguing at times. You're likely to experience muscle soreness at points, especially on days when you're trying new exercises or pushing yourself to a new level of strength. Also, if you take a few days off, you might find that getting back into the swing of things leaves you feeling sore.

Normal soreness should feel like an ache in your muscles, not pain in your joints. Your legs might feel heavy, and it might even take some maneuvering to get out of a chair after a really hard workout. Soreness is normal and part of the muscle-building process. However, if you are feeling extremely sore on a regular basis or immediately after every workout, you might be working too hard. If you feel joint pain or pain that radiates down a limb, seek medical attention to rule out an injury.

Check in with your feelings, too. If you're feeling stressed about working out, dreading it, or finding that it's making you upset, take a step back and evaluate your fitness plan. Your emotional health is important, too, and taking a few days off to bring your stress down could be just what you need to get back to enjoying your routine. If this doesn't help, it may be time to revisit your goal worksheet (page 9). As you remind yourself of your goals, consider taking a new approach to them, whether that means adopting a new routine or a different schedule, or inviting someone to join you in working out together for increased motivation and accountability.

No matter how successful your bodyweight training is, continue to listen to your body and look after all aspects of your health: exercise, nutrition, sleep, hydration, and emotional well-being.

chapter 3

EXERCISE TECHNIQUES

In this chapter, you'll learn a wide variety of movements. These will be combined in different ways to make up your twelve-week fitness journey. Take some time to familiarize yourself with the instructions and pictures of each movement before starting the program—this will help you approach the movements with confidence and accuracy. Pay close attention to the form described and refer to this section as often as needed until you are confident with each movement. The illustrations show optimal form and alignment. Although you'll want to emulate them, you should realize that not everybody will look the same doing an exercise. Read the instructions fully before starting—this will help you gain a deeper understanding of what you should be feeling during an exercise and what can be modified to suit your body best.

STRETCHING

Stretching is key to a well-rounded fitness program. It's best done regularly and has many benefits. Stretching can improve range of motion in joints that have tightened up from inactivity and undo some of the strain of suboptimal positions we often find ourselves in, such as hunching over a desk at work. A good stretch also can feel very relaxing after a challenging workout or strenuous day at the home or office—it's even a great way to start the day! Stretching can help improve flexibility with time and consistency; note that it will take at least three to four weeks to see a visible increase in range of motion.

The stretches described in this chapter are called **static stretches**, which are usually recommended for after your workout. Static stretches are isolated stretches that you hold in place while the muscle fibers slowly relax under the tension. You don't want to do static stretches on cold, inactive muscles. Rather, these kinds of stretches are most effective after your body has warmed up from movement.

You'll want to hold these stretches for at least thirty seconds to give the muscles time to relax and adapt. It's important not to force these or do them aggressively. Instead, while holding a static stretch, take deep, slow breaths, and use each exhale to gently move deeper into the stretch. The more you can relax, breathe, and enjoy the journey, the sweeter the rewards of stretching will be.

Wall Stretch for Chest

MUSCLES WORKED:
▶ **Pectoralis Major**
▶ **Pectoralis Minor**
▶ **Anterior Deltoids**

1. Stand at half-arm distance from the frame in a doorway, facing forward.

2. With your left arm outstretched at shoulder height, bend your elbow 90 degrees. Press the elevated forearm flat behind the doorframe and start to turn your body away from your left arm.

3. If desired, move your feet to facilitate more rotation and go deeper into the stretch. You should feel this stretch across the armpit of your left arm or in the front of your shoulder.

4. Hold for 30 seconds while breathing deeply.

5. Repeat on the opposite side.

6. To stretch a wider range of chest muscles, adjust the height of your elbow so it is higher than or below shoulder height.

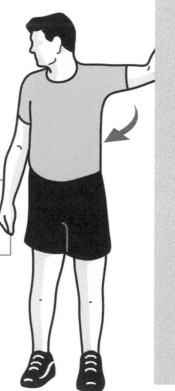

MODIFICATIONS/TIPS: If you feel numbness in your fingers, stop this stretch and approach it more slowly. Be sure to stay within a range of motion that feels good.

Standing Side Bends

MUSCLES WORKED:
- ▶ Quadratus Lumborum
- ▶ Latissimus Dorsi

1. Stand with your feet together and place your right hand on your hip. Cross your right leg in front of the left, then raise your left arm over your head.

2. Slowly bend your body to the right. Hold for 30 seconds while breathing deeply. Try to bend farther with each exhale. You should feel this stretch primarily in your rib cage and your waist. You also might feel it in your outer thighs and hips. Avoid collapsing into the shortened side, slumping forward, or leaning back.

3. Repeat steps 1 and 2 on the opposite side.

4. For a deeper stretch, try using the opposite arm to assist in pulling the raised arm farther into the bend.

> **MODIFICATIONS/TIPS:** If you find balancing with your feet crossed too challenging, try this stretch with your feet uncrossed and hip-width apart.

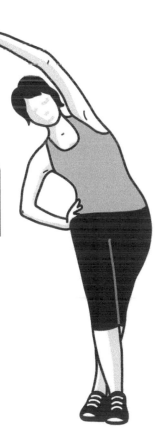

Wall Push for Full Back Body

MUSCLES WORKED:
- ▸ **Latissimus Dorsi**
- ▸ **Hamstrings**

1. Stand facing a wall 3 to 4 feet away. Stand with your feet wider than your hips and toes pointing straight ahead.

2. Lift your arms in front of you to shoulder height and lean forward until your hands reach the wall.

3. Keeping your hands at this height, push your hips back over your heels. You should feel this stretch primarily in your arms and shoulders. If you feel good there, you can walk your hands farther down the wall until they are at hip height.

4. Press your hands flat into the wall and push your butt farther back. This will facilitate a deeper stretch in your hamstrings. Hold for 30 seconds while breathing deeply.

5. For a deeper stretch, while keeping one hand on the wall, reach the other arm across the body toward the opposite ankle and hold for 10 seconds. Try both sides.

> **MODIFICATIONS/TIPS:** If you have shoulder pain, keep the arms a little higher than hip height, and make sure you aren't collapsing your shoulders.

Overhead Triceps Stretch

MUSCLES WORKED:
► **Triceps**

1. Stand with your feet hip-width apart and toes pointing straight ahead.

2. Lift your right arm straight up in the air, close to your body, and bend that elbow so your hand reaches behind your head.

3. Raise your left hand and place it on top of your right elbow. Allow your left hand to hold your right arm in place so you can stretch more. Work your right hand down so your fingers touch the middle of your upper spine. If you have tight triceps, you might only reach the bottom of your head.

4. Hold for 30 seconds while breathing deeply. You should feel this stretch primarily in your triceps, but also in the underarm area.

5. Return to the starting position and repeat on the other side.

6. For a deeper stretch, keeping one arm in the middle of the back, bring the opposite arm down and behind your back and try to reach the other hand from below. Grab that hand and hold it for 15 to 30 seconds.

> **MODIFICATIONS/TIPS:** If you feel pain in your shoulder, don't go deeper into this stretch.

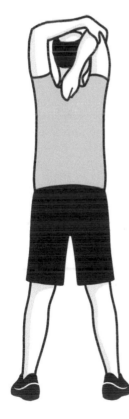

Standing Calf Stretch

MUSCLES WORKED:
▸ **Gastrocnemius**
▸ **Soleus**

1. Stand 3 feet away from a wall (a little farther if you are more than 6 feet tall).

2. Keeping both feet pointing straight at the wall, place your right foot a step closer and lean forward, placing your hands on the wall at shoulder height.

3. Press your weight forward into the wall as you simultaneously push your back heel down into the floor. You should feel a stretch in your calf on the back leg.

4. Hold for 30 seconds while breathing deeply.

5. Return to the starting position and repeat on the opposite side.

6. For a deeper stretch, keeping your feet in the same position, step back from the wall so you are standing more upright. Trying to keep your back foot on the floor, bend your back knee until you feel a stretch down toward your heel. Hold for 30 seconds.

MODIFICATIONS/TIPS: If you have Achilles tendinitis, this stretch should be avoided.

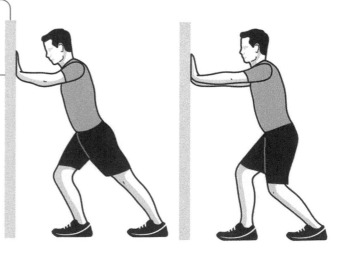

Standing Quadriceps Stretch

MUSCLES WORKED:
▸ **Quadriceps**

1. With your feet close together, stand near a countertop, chair, or steady surface to hold on to for stability.

2. Keeping your left leg straight, bend your right leg back and grasp your ankle with your right hand so it is held up behind you. If you can't reach your ankle, try looping a towel around your foot to hold it, or place your shin on a chair so your leg is straighter.

3. Use your right hand to assist in bending your knee more. Keep your thighs as parallel as you can while you stretch the right foot back. You should feel a stretch in your quadriceps muscle. Hold for 30 seconds while breathing deeply.

4. As you hold your position, focus on lengthening the front side of the body by contracting the glutes (butt muscles) to get taller. Try to keep your entire body tall and straight throughout the stretch.

5. Repeat with the opposite leg.

> **MODIFICATIONS/TIPS: If you feel knee pain in this stretch, you might be pulling too hard. Aim just to feel a gentle stretch in the quadriceps.**

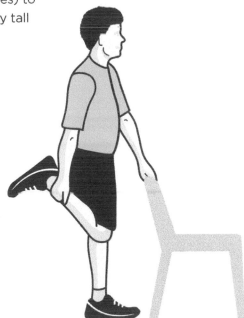

Standing Hamstring Stretch

MUSCLES WORKED:
► **Hamstrings**

1. Stand facing a step, box, or elevated platform, and place your right heel onto the surface, keeping both legs straight. If you must bend your knees or turn either of your feet out to keep the leg up, your step is too high. Keep your spine straight and hip bones facing straight ahead.

2. Bend forward at the hips, bringing your torso toward your right thigh and placing both hands comfortably down on that thigh. Hold for 30 seconds while breathing deeply.

3. Repeat with the opposite leg.

4. If you're able to maintain good balance, alignment, and straight legs while holding this stretch and desire a deeper stretch, flex the foot of your elevated leg so the toes are pulling back toward your torso. Try to touch your toes with one hand.

> **MODIFICATIONS/TIPS: Avoid resting your hands directly on your knee, which could strain it.**

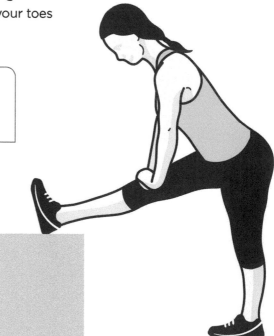

Butterfly Stretch

MUSCLES WORKED:
▶ **Adductors**

1. Come to a seated position on the ground. Sit up tall with the soles of your feet pressing into each other and your knees dropped to your sides. If this position is uncomfortable for you, you can sit on a folded towel, blanket, or pillow.

2. Place your hands on your feet or ankles.

3. Take a deep breath and lengthen your spine so you feel lifted above your hips, then lean forward slightly until you feel a gentle stretch along the inside of your thighs. Hold this for 30 seconds.

4. For a deeper stretch, prop some towels under your knees so you can relax more and hold the stretch for longer.

> **MODIFICATIONS/TIPS: Use caution if you have a knee or groin injury.**

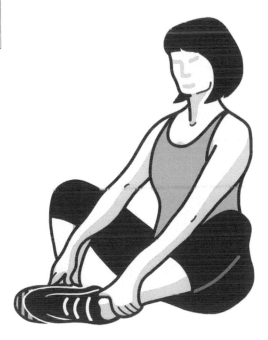

Figure 4 Stretch

MUSCLES WORKED:
- ▶ Gluteus Medius
- ▶ Piriformis

1. Lie flat on your back with your knees bent and feet on the ground.

2. Cross your right ankle over your left thigh.

3. Reach through your legs with both hands to clasp them together behind your left thigh.

4. Holding this position, lift both feet off the ground and pull both legs in toward your chest. Keep your head and neck relaxed on the ground. Hold for 30 seconds while breathing deeply. You should feel a deep stretch in the outer right hip.

5. Repeat on the other side.

6. For a deeper stretch, flex the foot of the crossed leg and open your hip more by pressing with your hand on your top knee so it gently goes farther out to the side.

MODIFICATIONS/TIPS: Make sure to keep your back flat on the ground.

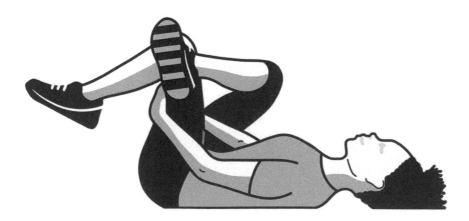

CORE

The core is the center of the body and the foundation upon which we build all our strength. A strong core is essential for bodyweight training to be safe and effective. It can also improve posture and alleviate or prevent chronic lower back pain.

The major muscles of the core move and stabilize your spine—these muscles include the rectus abdominis, internal and external obliques, spinal erectors, diaphragm, pelvic floor muscles, and transverse abdominis. Some other important muscles that have an impact on core function include the latissimus dorsi, hip flexors, gluteus maximus, and adductors.

The transverse abdominis is a very deep core muscle that lies underneath your rectus abdominis and obliques and wraps all the way around your spine. When the transverse abdominis contracts, it hugs the spine like a corset. If you can imagine someone was about to punch you in the stomach and you stood still but braced your abs for the impact, you would feel your transverse abdominis contracting. Learning to engage this muscle and strengthening it with core training will keep your midsection tight and sturdy to support exercise.

When doing bodyweight training focused on the core, it's helpful to keep this image of a corset tightening around your midsection as you exhale so you experience 360-degree activation of your transverse abdominis.

Low Plank

MUSCLES WORKED:
- ▶ **Rectus Abdominis**
- ▶ **Transverse Abdominis**
- ▶ **Spinal Extensors**

1. Lie on your stomach on the floor, then lift your body so you are supported on your forearms and your toes. Position your elbows directly under your shoulders, with your feet flexed and slightly wider than hip-width apart and your torso parallel to the floor with a neutral curve in your spine.

2. Hold this position for up to 60 seconds while focusing on your breath. Inhale deeply through your nose and feel the air filling your belly and 360 degrees around your spine. Exhale slowly and feel your belly button pulling up against gravity and your abdominal muscles tightening around your middle.

> MODIFICATIONS/TIPS: **If your back feels strained or you notice your lower spine is sinking with your butt sticking out, decrease intensity by doing an Incline Plank: Find a couch or ottoman to create an elevated platform that can support your upper-body weight.**

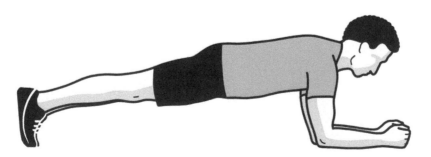

Basic Crunch

MUSCLES WORKED:
► **Rectus Abdominis**

1. Lie on your back with your knees bent, legs hip-width apart, and feet flat on the floor. You can lay a mat or towel under your spine.

2. Place your hands behind your head and interlace your fingers to support your head and neck. Tuck your chin down slightly, keeping some space between your chin and chest.

3. Curl up and forward, lifting your head and shoulders slightly off the ground. Exhale as you crunch and reach the point where the tops of your abs are squeezing tight but the bottom of your rib cage is still touching the ground. Don't go into a full sit-up. Inhale as you release the crunch, and return your head to the floor.

4. For a more challenging crunch, lift your feet and bring legs up to a 90-degree angle as you do the exercise or squeeze a pillow between your thighs as you crunch.

> MODIFICATIONS/TIPS: **If you're a beginner, you might feel some strain in your neck. That's normal while you are building up strength in this exercise. Try to move smoothly and not to jerk up too hard or fast.**

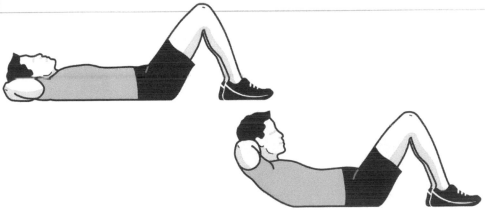

Reverse Crunch

MUSCLES WORKED:
► **Rectus Abdominis**

1. Lie on your back with your legs in the air and bent at a 90-degree angle. Keep your knees together, but not squeezing tight.

2. Place both hands on the ground next to your butt or, if you have a sensitive back, tilt your pelvis up a little and place your hands underneath your butt.

3. Keeping your head, neck, and shoulders on the floor, lift your butt off the ground by crunching just the lower half of your spine. Aim to lift your butt only 2 to 4 inches off the floor, making sure your lower body lifts toward the ceiling and doesn't roll back over your shoulders.

4. Control a slow descent as your butt returns to the ground.

5. Exhale as your legs go upward, and inhale as you come down.

> MODIFICATIONS/TIPS: **For an easier version, place your hands behind your head and perform a Basic Crunch (page 37) while simultaneously doing the Reverse Crunch.**

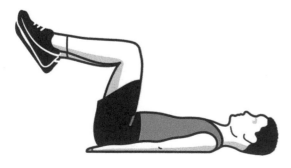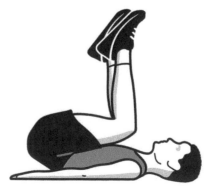

Dead Bug

1. Lie on your back with your arms straight up in the air over your shoulders, fingertips pointing up at the ceiling and your legs bent at a 90-degree angle with your knees directly over your hips.

2. Without changing your arm and leg position, engage your core by pressing your lower spine flat into the floor. You should feel your abdominals working to hold this position.

3. Keeping your lower back pressing into the floor, slowly lower your left leg downward and your right arm overhead so they are both extended and hovering a few inches off the floor. Hold this position for 5 seconds.

4. Slowly return to the starting position, and repeat with opposite limbs.

5. To get the most out of this exercise, inhale as you lower your limbs and exhale as you return to your starting position.

MODIFICATIONS/TIPS: If you feel like your lower back keeps popping up, shorten your range of motion and keep working on this exercise to build a good foundation.

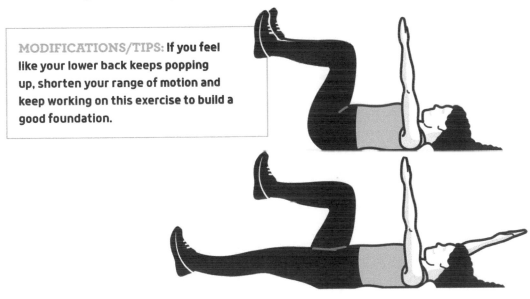

Side Plank

MUSCLES WORKED:
- ► Quadratus Lumborum
- ► Internal Obliques
- ► External Obliques
- ► Transverse Abdominis

1. Lie on your side with your forearm resting on the ground, elbow directly underneath your shoulder and legs stacked with knees slightly bent.

2. Press your hips up in the air so your knees and forearm are your base of support.

3. Your top hand can be on the side of your hip. For a more challenging version, raise your top arm up in the air in a straight line from your top arm's fingertips to your bottom arm's elbow, running perpendicular to the floor. Make sure the elbow on the floor lines up with your shoulder.

4. Hold the lifted position for up to 30 seconds.

5. Turn over and repeat on the opposite side.

6. Once you can hold this position for 30 seconds, try straightening your legs in the starting position, placing one foot in front of the other and pushing up on the sides of your feet instead of your knees.

MODIFICATIONS/TIPS: If you have a history of shoulder injury, this is an important exercise to master, but you may have to take it slow. If you feel shoulder pain, check your alignment and focus on creating space in the shoulder joint as you lift.

Scapula Push-Up

MUSCLES WORKED:
► **Serratus Anterior**

1. Stand facing an elevated step, sturdy coffee table, or low countertop. Place your hands shoulder-width apart on the surface and walk your feet back so you are leaning against the surface with straight arms. Make sure your wrists are directly under your shoulders. Your heels will be lifted off the ground, so you are on your toes.

2. From this plank position, keep your elbows straight as you inhale and sink into your shoulder blades. Then exhale as you press the shoulder blades as far apart as you can. Keep your body in the plank position. The only visible movement will be in your scapula (shoulder blades).

MODIFICATIONS/TIPS: **Although your arms should be straight in this exercise, make sure you are not hyperextending your elbow joints or overstretching your wrists against the surface. If you feel weak in these joints, you can work on the scapula from your forearms in the Low Plank position.**

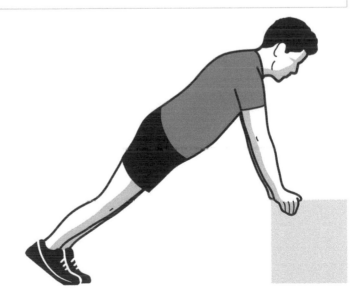

High Plank

MUSCLES WORKED:
- ▶ **Transverse Abdominis**
- ▶ **Rectus Abdominis**

1. Lie on your stomach on the floor, then lift your body so you are supported on your hands and toes.

2. Position your wrists directly under your shoulders, with your hands pointing straight ahead and your fingers spread, feet flexed, and torso parallel to the floor with a neutral curve in your spine.

3. Hold this position for up to 60 seconds while focusing on your breath.

4. Inhale deeply through your nose and feel the air fill your belly and 360 degrees around your spine. Exhale slowly and feel your belly button pull up against gravity and your abdominal muscles tighten around your middle.

MODIFICATIONS/TIPS: **If you have wrist pain, you may need to build strength slowly in this position. You can also put your hands into fists to avoid stressing the wrist joint.**

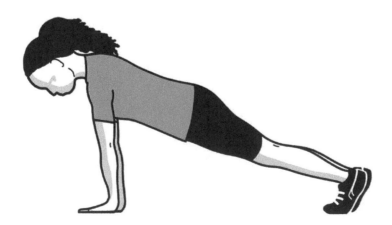

Rotating Side Plank

MUSCLES WORKED:
- ▶ Quadratus Lumborum
- ▶ Internal Obliques
- ▶ External Obliques
- ▶ Transverse Abdominis

1. Lie on your side with your elbow directly underneath your shoulder and your legs stacked with your knees slightly bent.

2. Press your hips up in the air so your knees and forearm support you.

3. Raise your top arm up in the air in a straight line from your top fingertips to your bottom elbow, running perpendicular to the floor. Make sure your bottom elbow lines up with your shoulder and doesn't slide up by your ear.

4. In this lifted position, twist your top arm far enough underneath your bottom armpit to feel your midsection working, and then rotate open again. Try to stay lifted as you perform the rotation, with your hips remaining lifted and your shoulders supported. Repeat the sequence for the desired number of repetitions.

5. Turn over and repeat on the opposite side.

6. To increase the challenge, try this with straight legs.

MODIFICATIONS/TIPS:
If you have a history of shoulder injury, this is an important exercise to master, but you may have to take it slow. If you feel shoulder pain, check your alignment and focus on creating space in the shoulder joint as you lift.

UPPER BODY

Upper-body strength is essential for keeping the body in balance as we age. Our arms, back, chest, and shoulders help hold us erect and in good posture and are responsible for all our pushing and pulling tasks. A strong upper body will make those heavy grocery bags feel a lot lighter!

When focusing on upper body in your bodyweight training, you'll find that almost every exercise requires your core to get involved. Engaging your core will keep you grounded and stable as you move your arms through resistance and help you get stronger faster. Upper-body bodyweight training exercises integrate many muscles at once, rather than a single muscle in isolation. This makes these exercises beneficial on a broader level than using weight machines in a gym. Because you are engaging more muscles, you'll get a greater metabolic effect.

Joint pain is always something to be mindful of, but it can be especially prevalent with shoulder and elbow exercises. Some overuse injuries, like shoulder impingement or tennis elbow, can be aggravated by certain arm movements, so consult an orthopedist or physical therapist beforehand if you have a history of this kind of pain or injury.

Triceps Dip Bent Leg

MUSCLES WORKED:

▶ **Triceps**

▶ **Pectoralis Major**

▶ **Serratus Anterior**

▶ **Trapezius**

1. Stand and place your hands slightly wider than shoulder-width apart on the edge of a sturdy chair or step behind you. Lower your hips to the level of your hands, putting your feet out slightly in front of you hip-width apart, with your knees bent and feet on the floor (or heels only for a greater challenge). Your butt should be pitched just past the edge of the chair or step.

2. Keeping your spine upright, lower yourself until your elbows are bent close to 90 degrees.

3. Push back up to straight arms. Try to use only arms, not legs, in pushing up.

4. For a more advanced version, after you have straightened your arms, press your shoulder blades farther down your spine so you are even higher up. You should feel this in your lower trapezius muscle.

> **MODIFICATIONS/TIPS:** Avoid this exercise if you have shoulder impingement or are prone to shoulder injury. If you have sensitive shoulders, focus on keeping your spine upright as you lower yourself, and don't lower yourself all the way to 90 degrees at the elbow; stay higher.

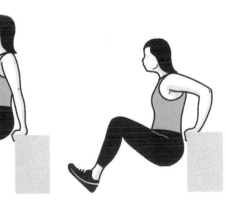

Triceps Dip Straight Leg

MUSCLES WORKED:
- ▶ **Triceps**
- ▶ **Pectoralis Major**
- ▶ **Serratus Anterior**
- ▶ **Trapezius**

1. Stand and place your hands just slightly wider than shoulder-width apart on the edge of a chair or step behind you. Lower your hips to the level of your hands, putting your feet out in front of you with straight legs and flexed feet. Your hands and heels will be the two points of contact. Your butt should be pitched just past the edge of the chair or step.

2. Keeping your spine upright, lower yourself until your elbows are bent close to 90 degrees.

3. Push back up to straight arms.

4. For a more advanced version, use a second chair or step to place your heels up on.

> **MODIFICATIONS/TIPS:** Avoid this exercise if you have shoulder impingement.

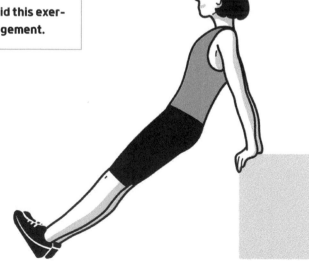

Climbing Plank

MUSCLES WORKED:

- ▶ **Triceps**
- ▶ **Anterior Deltoids**
- ▶ **Transverse Abdominis**
- ▶ **Serratus Anterior**

1. Begin in a **Low Plank** position (page 36).

2. Press into the ground with your right arm and straighten it, positioning your wrist directly under your shoulder. Follow with your left arm so you are up in a **High Plank** (page 42) on your hands and toes.

3. Lower your right side back down onto your forearm and follow with the left. You should feel the effort in your triceps and abdominals.

4. Repeat the sequence but lead with your left arm.

> **MODIFICATIONS/TIPS:** For lower intensity, instead of coming up to a full **High Plank**, straighten one arm only and hold it up for a few seconds before going back to **Low Plank**. Switch arms. As you work on this, place more weight on the straightened arm each time until you feel confident you can support yourself enough to progress to the full **Climbing Plank**.

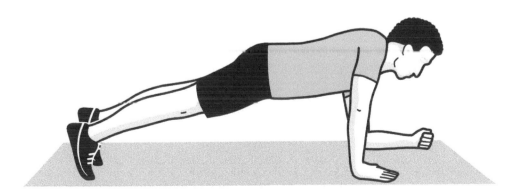

Side-Lying Triceps Press

MUSCLES WORKED:
- ▶ **Triceps**
- ▶ **Middle Deltoids**

1. Lie on your side with your knees bent and legs stacked. Place your bottom arm across your chest so your hand is holding the opposite shoulder. Place the other hand on the floor about 6 inches away from your chest.

2. Press your top arm until fully straightened, lifting your whole upper body sideways but keeping your hips and knees anchored on the floor. Lower yourself back to the floor and immediately repeat without resting between repetitions. You should feel the effort on the outside of your upper arm, triceps, and top of your shoulder.

3. Turn over and repeat on the opposite side.

> **MODIFICATIONS/TIPS:** Try to keep your head facing forward without twisting your neck during this exercise.

Right-Angle Arm Twist

MUSCLES WORKED:
► **Rotator Cuff**
► **Biceps**

1. Stand with your arms bent at 90-degree angles, out to the sides from your shoulders, palms facing down.

2. Keeping your upper arms in place at the level of your shoulder, rotate your lower arms upward so your hands lift to the level of your head, maintaining the 90-degree bend at the elbow.

3. Return to the starting position, keeping tension in your back and biceps.

MODIFICATIONS/TIPS: **To go deeper, do this exercise standing with your back against a wall. When your forearms and hands reach the wall, press hard into the wall for a few seconds before returning to starting position.**

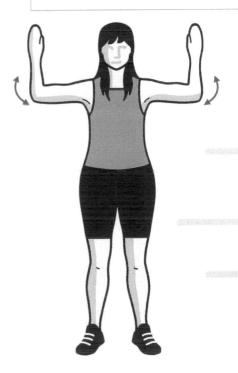

Prone Overhead Shoulder Press

MUSCLES WORKED:
► **Anterior Deltoids**
► **Middle Deltoids**
► **Posterior Deltoids**
► **Spinal Erectors**
► **Trapezius, Rhomboids**

1. Lie on your stomach with your feet and knees together and the tops of your feet touching the floor. Bend your arms next to your sides with your hands at shoulder level and elbows next to your rib cage.

2. Look up slightly and lift your upper body about 6 inches off the floor, keeping your lower body anchored to the floor. You should feel your middle back muscles engage.

3. Keeping your arms at the height of your ears, extend them overhead, parallel to the floor. You will feel a stretch on the outside of your armpits and your rib cage.

4. Return your hands to your shoulders and your elbows to your sides. Keep your upper body lifted between repetitions.

MODIFICATIONS/TIPS:
You can build up your strength in this exercise by lowering your upper body back to the floor between each repetition and esting your head to one side.

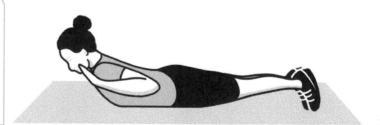

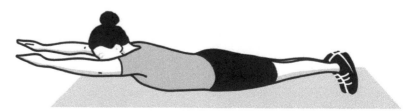

High Plank to Downward Dog

MUSCLES WORKED:
- ▶ **Anterior Deltoids**
- ▶ **Middle Deltoids**
- ▶ **Transverse Abdominis**

1. Start in a **High Plank** position (page 42), but on your hands and toes. If you're double-jointed or very flexible in your elbows, make sure they are not hyperextended while performing your plank.

2. Leading with your hips, stick your butt up in the air, press your heels back into the ground, and push your chest forward slightly through your shoulders. Your body will be in the shape of a triangle with the floor—this is **Downward Dog**. Keep your spine neutral.

3. Hold this position for 3 seconds, then rock your bodyweight forward onto your toes and return your hips and shoulders to the plank position.

4. For more of a challenge, instead of counting seconds in each position, count 3 breaths. Inhale through your nose and let your belly fill with air, then exhale through your mouth and draw your belly button in toward your spine, tightening around your transverse abdominis.

MODIFICATIONS/TIPS: In High Plank, be careful not to arch your back. In Downward Dog, keep the scapula engaged, and don't overstretch your chest by letting it collapse too deeply between your shoulders.

Inverted Scapula Press-Up

MUSCLES WORKED:
- ▶ **Anterior Deltoids**
- ▶ **Middle Deltoids**
- ▶ **Serratus Anterior**
- ▶ **Trapezius**

1. Begin in a tabletop position on hands and knees, with your hands and arms under your shoulders and your knees hip-width apart and a sturdy chair, step, or platform behind you.

2. Extend your legs and put your feet on the seat of the chair. Hike your hips up high so they are over your shoulders, keeping arms straight. You will be upside-down.

3. Keeping your arms straight, lower slightly into the shoulder blades and then push them apart as your whole body lifts a few inches. You will feel like you are doing an upside-down shoulder shrug.

MODIFICATIONS/TIPS: **Avoid this exercise if you have vertigo or a fear of falling. Make sure you are comfortable performing the High Plank to Downward Dog (page 51) and Prone Overhead Shoulder Press (page 50) before attempting this exercise.**

Spiderman Push-Up

MUSCLES WORKED:
- ▶ **Pectoralis Major**
- ▶ **Anterior Deltoids**
- ▶ **Triceps**
- ▶ **Rectus Abdominis**

1. Begin in a **High Plank** position (page 42).

2. Move your right hand 12 inches in front of your shoulder and draw your left knee up to the outside of your left elbow, letting your left toes touch the floor. Bend both elbows and lower your body until your upper arms and torso are at elbow level.

3. Exhale as you straighten your arms and do a push-up. Bring the right arm and left leg back to **High Plank** position.

4. Repeat the sequence but with the opposite limbs.

5. For more of a challenge, keep the foot of the moving leg in the air as you do the push-up.

> **MODIFICATIONS/TIPS:** For an easier version, go onto your knees and do an uneven arm push-up, alternating the arm in front and the arm that stays at your side.

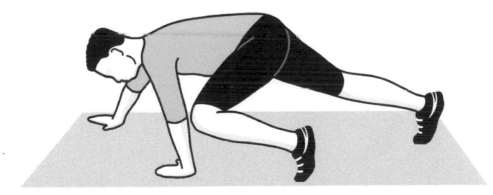

Plank Overhead Reaches

MUSCLES WORKED:
- ▸ **Posterior Deltoids**
- ▸ **Transverse Abdominis**

1. Begin in a **High Plank** position (page 42).

2. Raise your right arm in line with your shoulder while turning that hand so your thumb side is facing upward. Hold it there for 3 seconds. Keep your torso parallel to the floor with your hips facing down.

3. Lower your arm back to **High Plank** and switch arms to repeat the sequence.

4. As you raise your arm away from your center of gravity, your body will want to follow it. Use the muscles in your waist and rib cage to stop the twist from happening and keep your torso parallel to the floor.

> MODIFICATIONS/TIPS: For an easier version, begin on your hands and knees in a tabletop position, your hands and arms under your shoulders and your knees hip-width apart. Engage your core as you raise your arm in line with your shoulder while turning that hand so the thumb is pointing up at the ceiling. Hold for 3 seconds. The three legs of your "table" on the floor should remain in the same position. Don't collapse into your hips or shoulders. Return the raised arm to tabletop and alternate sides.

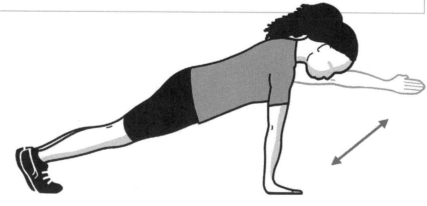

Prayer Pulse

MUSCLES WORKED:
► **Pectoralis Major**

1. Standing with your legs hip-width apart, bring your arms straight out to the sides at shoulder height. Bend your elbows to a 90-degree angle with your forearms up, palms flat and facing forward.

2. Keeping the elbows bent at 90 degrees, bring your arms toward each other until you can press your palms and elbows together. Try to keep your upper arms at shoulder height throughout the movement. Return to the starting position.

3. Exhale while you are pressing, and inhale as you open your chest and release the contraction.

MODIFICATIONS/TIPS: **For a more advanced version, while holding the pressed position, move your arms straight up and down, keeping your elbows between the height of your chin and your nose. As you do, don't let any space come between your forearms.**

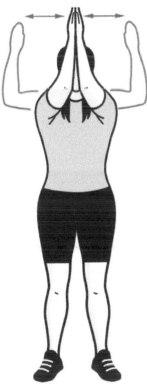

Push-Up

MUSCLES WORKED:
- ▶ **Pectoralis Major**
- ▶ **Triceps**
- ▶ **Anterior Deltoids**

1. Begin in a **High Plank** position (page 42) with your hands placed slightly wider than shoulder-width apart.

2. Inhale as you lower your body by bending your elbows to a 90-degree angle. You should feel a stretch across your chest and burning in your biceps. If your shoulders feel strong, you can lower past 90 degrees and touch your chest to the floor.

3. Exhale as you straighten your arms and push up back to starting position.

> MODIFICATIONS/TIPS: **Push-ups require a lot of arm strength, but if your plank position isn't solid, you can strain your back. Make sure you can maintain a neutral spine as you perform this exercise. If you notice your back arching, take a rest or finish on your knees. Don't forget to breathe!**

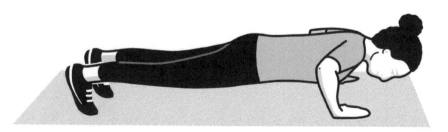

Push-Up to Side Plank

MUSCLES WORKED:
- ► Pectoralis Major
- ► Anterior Deltoids
- ► Triceps
- ► Transverse Abdominis
- ► Quadratus Lumborum

1. Begin in a **High Plank** position (page 42) with your hands placed slightly wider than shoulder-width apart.

2. Inhale as you lower your body by bending your elbows to a 90-degree angle.

3. On your exhale, push up and straighten your arms. As you do, shift your weight to your left arm and push your right arm off the ground, reaching that hand up toward the sky and opening the chest to face right. As you open your right arm, let your feet roll to the side so your whole body is facing right. Keep your hips in line with your shoulders.

4. Return your right arm and body to the **High Plank** position and repeat steps 2 and 3 on the opposite side.

5. For more of a challenge, when you reach your arm up, take a moment to stack your feet and challenge your body to balance sideways on this narrower base of support.

MODIFICATIONS/TIPS: **If you are a beginner, you can do this exercise on your knees.**

Exercise Techniques   57

Eccentric Push-Up to Cobra

MUSCLES WORKED:
▸ **Pectoralis Major**
▸ **Triceps**
▸ **Posterior Deltoids**
▸ **Spinal Erectors**

1. Begin in a **High Plank** position (page 42).

2. Bending your elbows, lower your body as slowly as possible all the way to the floor. This should feel like a slow motion push-up all the way down. Allow your chest and stomach to reach the floor at the same time.

3. Press your legs into the floor and lift your entire upper body off the floor, along with your arms. Arch your upper back and squeeze your shoulder blades together. This will look like the **Cobra** (page 63) except with your feet hip-width apart. Hold this position for a few seconds.

4. Slowly lower your upper body back to the floor. Engage your arms and legs to push back up into the **High Plank** position.

MODIFICATIONS/TIPS:
The most important part of this exercise is lowering (step 2) and doing the Cobra (step 3). If you need to "cheat" rising from the floor back into your plank position, that's okay–you will still build strength doing the first 3 steps. You can also do step 2 on your knees.

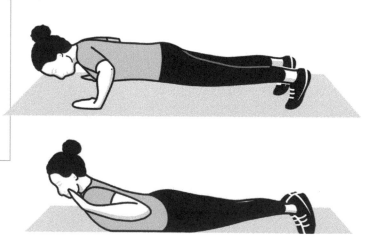

Side-Walking Plank

MUSCLES WORKED:
- ▶ **Pectoralis Major**
- ▶ **Pectoralis Minor**
- ▶ **Triceps**
- ▶ **Transverse Abdominis**

1. Begin in a **High Plank** position (page 42).

2. Move your right hand 6 inches out to the right while simultaneously moving your right foot 6 inches to the right. Shift your weight over to the right arm and leg as you move your left arm and left leg simultaneously to the right 6 inches. Your body will once again be in the **High Plank** position. Continue repetitions by stepping to the right 3 or 4 more times.

3. As your body moves, keep your hips level and avoid hiking them up in the air.

4. Repeat step 2 in the opposite direction.

> **MODIFICATIONS/TIPS:** If you can't move your arm and leg simultaneously, start by moving your hand, and then follow with the same-side leg before moving the other hand: right foot, right hand, left foot, left hand, and vice versa.

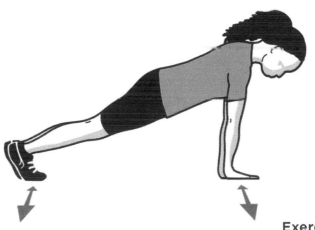

Low Plank 90-Degree Pec Fly

MUSCLES WORKED:
- ▸ Pectoralis Major
- ▸ Serratus Anterior
- ▸ Posterior Deltoid
- ▸ Transverse Abdominis

1. Begin in a **Low Plank** position (page 36).

2. Press your left forearm firmly into the floor. Keeping the 90-degree bend in your right elbow, lift your right arm out to shoulder height, parallel to the floor. Try to keep your hips from twisting and keep your torso facing the floor as you move your arm to the side.

3. Return your right arm to **Low Plank** position, but don't put weight back on it. Repeat the movement.

4. Do the desired number of repetitions, then repeat the entire sequence on the other side.

MODIFICATIONS/TIPS: **If you are a beginner, do the plank from your knees.**

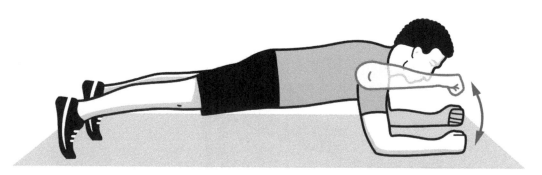

Bird Dog

MUSCLES WORKED:

▶ **Spinal Erectors**

▶ **Transverse Abdominis**

▶ **Gluteus Maximus**

▶ **Posterior Deltoids**

1. Begin in a tabletop position on your hands and knees, with your hands and arms under your shoulders and your knees hip-width apart. Engage your abdominals and maintain a neutral spine.

2. Raise your right arm in front of you, with the thumb side facing upward, and left leg behind you simultaneously, keeping your shoulders and hips parallel to the floor. Stretch your left leg out long, straightening the knee fully. Point your right thumb upward.

3. Hold this extended position for a few seconds. Keep your head in line with the rest of your spine and don't extend your chin too far up or down.

4. Return to the tabletop position and repeat with the opposite limbs.

> MODIFICATIONS/TIPS: **If you have sensitive knees, you can place some padding underneath.**

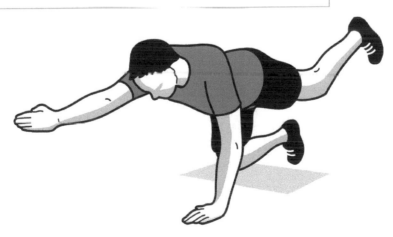

Lat Slides

MUSCLES WORKED:
- ▶ **Latissimus Dorsi**
- ▶ **Rectus Abdominis**

1. For this exercise you will need a hard floor and a small towel.

2. Begin in a tabletop position on hands and knees with your hands slightly wider than shoulder-width apart. Place the towel underneath your knees.

3. Keeping your arms straight and hands planted, slide your knees backward, pulling your shoulders in the same direction. Your body will lower as you slide back. Go as far back as your arms will allow.

4. Engaging your back muscles and keeping your abdominals tight, with straight arms, pull your body back to the starting position. You should feel a pull underneath your armpits and a tightening of your abdominals near the top of your rib cage.

> MODIFICATIONS/TIPS: **For a more advanced version, begin in a High Plank (page 42) position with your feet on the towel instead of your knees. It takes a lot of total body strength and control to lower your body close to the floor, so even if you can go back only a few inches, make sure the movement is happening from your shoulders.**

Cobra

MUSCLES WORKED:
- ► **Posterior Deltoids**
- ► **Latissimus Dorsi**
- ► **Rhomboids**

1. Lie on your stomach with your arms bent by your sides. Your hands should be approximately 6 inches out from and at the height of your shoulders. Keep your legs tight together with the tops of your feet facing the floor and your heels touching each other.

2. Lift your upper body and arms off the floor while squeezing your shoulder blades toward each other. Keeping your legs on the floor, squeeze your inner thighs and glutes tight to anchor your lower body and feet to the floor. Keep your gaze in line with the movement of your upper body. Your arm muscles should remain engaged.

3. Hold this position for a few seconds before softly returning your upper body to the ground.

> **MODIFICATIONS/TIPS:** For a more advanced version, instead of bending your arms at the elbows by your sides, keep your arms straight out from your shoulders, forming a T-shape as you lift your upper body, keeping your arm muscles engaged as you rise.

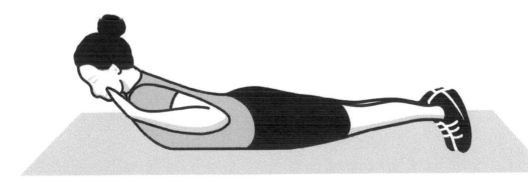

Prone Swimmer

MUSCLES WORKED:
- ▶ Spinal Erectors
- ▶ Latissimus Dorsi
- ▶ Gluteus Maximus

1. Lie on your stomach with your legs outstretched slightly wider than your hips and arms stretched overhead at the same width apart as the legs. Keep your palms down with your fingers together. Point your toes.

2. Lift your right arm and your left leg as high as you can. Keep your leg straight at the knee so the lower-body movement comes from your hip. Keep your hip bones pressing into the ground so your weight doesn't shift to any one side.

3. Lower your right arm and left leg back to starting position, and repeat with the opposite limbs.

> MODIFICATIONS/TIPS: **Lift your gaze to the level of your elbow so your head extends up slightly. Avoid looking up too high and straining your neck.**

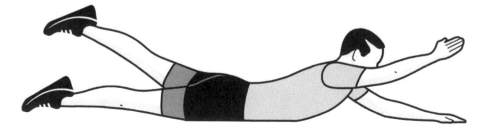

Superman

MUSCLES WORKED:
- ▶ Spinal Erectors
- ▶ Latissimus Dorsi
- ▶ Gluteus Maximus

1. Lie on your stomach with your legs outstretched slightly wider than your hips and your arms stretched overhead at the same width apart as the legs. Keep your palms down with your fingers together. Point your toes.

2. Lift up your straight legs, straight arms, and head. Keep your hip bones anchored to the ground.

3. Lift your gaze to the level of your elbow so your head extends up slightly. Avoid looking too high up and straining your neck. You should feel your glutes squeezing as you lift your legs and your upper back engaging as you lift your arms.

4. Hold for 3 seconds, then softly return to the ground.

MODIFICATIONS/TIPS: **The lower-body portion of this exercise will be most effective with a very straight knee. Engage your quadriceps muscle in the front of the thigh to make your leg one long line extending from the hip.**

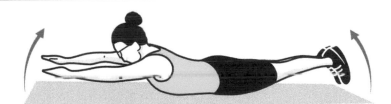

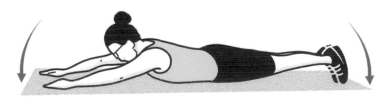

LOWER BODY

The muscles in the lower body are large and have many blood vessels running through them; therefore, bodyweight exercises that target the lower body often elevate the heart rate, and you might feel like you're doing a cardiovascular exercise. Lower-body exercises burn a lot of calories, strengthen your heart, and improve balance and agility. You'll feel many benefits every day from working out this area, such as when climbing stairs, walking up a hill, running to catch a bus, and even getting out of a low chair.

The big, dynamic movements of lower-body exercises such as squats and lunges are very important for building strength and power in your quadriceps, hamstrings, and gastrocnemius and soleus (calves). But the smaller, more isolated exercises that target your adductors (inner thighs), abductors (outer thighs), and glutes (butt) are equally important for building stability to protect your hips, knees, and ankles when performing the larger movements.

If you are new to lower-body exercise, you might feel weakness or a little strain in your knees when you begin. As you strengthen the quadriceps and hamstring muscles after a few workouts, that weak feeling should go away.

Side-Lying Leg Raises

MUSCLES WORKED:
- ▸ **Gluteus Medius**
- ▸ **Gluteus Minimus**

1. Lie on your side with your bottom leg bent and top leg completely straight. Keep the foot on your top leg flexed. Let your bottom arm prop up your head or cradle it on the floor and your top hand rest on the floor in front of your torso.

2. Lift your top leg as high as you can, keeping your knee pointing straight ahead and making sure not to rotate your hip open.

3. Slowly bring your top leg back to starting position, and repeat the movement without resting the leg between repetitions. Keep the moving leg engaged and completely straight throughout the movement.

4. Turn over and repeat on the opposite side.

> MODIFICATIONS/TIPS: **Don't worry about how high you can lift your leg; instead, think about having control over the movement throughout the entire range of motion.**

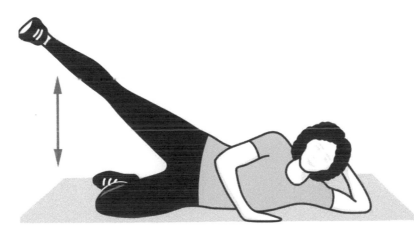

Side-Lying Inner-Thigh Leg Raises

MUSCLE WORKED:
▸ **Adductors**

1. Lie on your side with your top leg bent behind your bottom leg, and the foot of the top leg resting on the floor. Keep your bottom leg completely straight with the foot flexed. Let your bottom arm prop up your head or cradle it on the floor and let your top hand rest on the floor in front of your torso.

2. Lift your bottom leg as high off the floor as you can, keeping your leg straight and the knee pointing forward. Avoid rolling over onto your bottom glute or your back. The control of movement is the key to feeling this exercise in the right place. You should feel this in your inner thighs and groin muscles.

3. Slowly bring your bottom leg back to starting position, and repeat the sequence without resting the leg between repetitions. Turn over and repeat on the opposite side.

4. For more of a challenge, at the top of the range of motion, add an inner-thigh twist by turning the bottom leg inward and up.

MODIFICATIONS/TIPS: **If you find it difficult to lift your bottom leg, you can push a little bit with your top arm to assist yourself until your legs get stronger.**

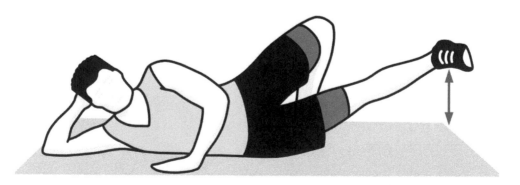

Clamshells

MUSCLES WORKED:
- ▶ **Gluteus Medius**
- ▶ **Gluteus Minimus**
- ▶ **Piriformis**

1. Lie on your side with your legs stacked and bent to a 90-degree angle at your hips and knees. Let your bottom arm cradle your head on the floor and your top hand rest on the floor in front of your torso.

2. Keeping the insides of your feet touching, open your knees as far as you can. Control the movement and bring your legs back to a stacked position. Repeat the sequence without resting between repetitions.

3. Turn over and repeat on the opposite side.

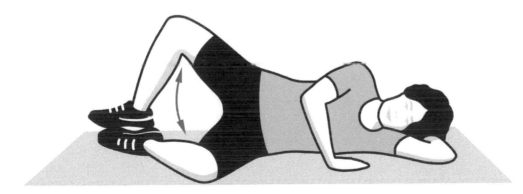

Lateral Lunge

MUSCLES WORKED:
▸ **Gluteus Maximus**
▸ **Adductors**
▸ **Outer Thighs**
▸ **Quadriceps**
▸ **Hamstrings**

1. Stand with your legs together, feet pointing straight ahead and hands by your sides. Keeping both feet pointing straight ahead, take a wide step out to the side with your left leg and bend your left hip back in a single-leg squat position. Keep your right leg straight. You will feel a stretch in your right inner thigh. Reach across with your right hand to touch the toes on your left foot.

2. Push off your left leg to return the legs together. Repeat the movement starting with the right leg.

3. Keep your spine straight and avoid rounding it, even as you reach down for the opposite toe.

4. For more of a challenge, start balanced on one foot. Perform your lateral lunge and then return to your balance.

MODIFICATIONS/TIPS: **If you are a beginner or have weak knees, start with your feet a full leg's length apart. Instead of stepping, glide your hips into the** Lateral Lunge **position. If your inner thighs are very tight, warm up with some jogging in place or jumping jacks before doing this exercise.**

Curtsy Lunge

MUSCLES WORKED:
- ► **Gluteus Maximus**
- ► **Adductors**
- ► **Outer Thighs**
- ► **Quadriceps**
- ► **Hamstrings**

1. Stand with your legs hip-width apart. Cross your left leg behind your right leg, and bend your knees and hips simultaneously in a "curtsy," putting some weight on your left toes and ball of the foot.

2. From the curtsy position, bring your left leg back to the starting position. During these movements, focus on posture and control rather than trying to get deeper in your hips and knees. Make sure the knee on the front leg is pointing straight ahead and is lined up with the toes on that leg. If desired for balance, you can hold on to a chair in front of you or something sturdy for support.

3. Repeat in the opposite position.

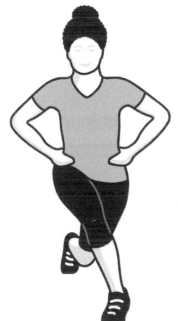

MODIFICATIONS/TIPS: **If your hips are very tight, warm them up by doing a few minutes of sideways-walking "grapevines." Move laterally as you quickly alternate crossing one leg in front and behind the other. Avoid the Curtsy Lunge and this warm-up if you've had a hip replacement.**

Lateral Bounds

MUSCLES WORKED:

- ▶ **Gluteus Maximus**
- ▶ **Adductors**
- ▶ **Outer Thighs**
- ▶ **Quadriceps**
- ▶ **Hamstrings**
- ▶ **Internal and External Obliques**

1. Stand on your right leg with your left leg off the ground. Propel yourself to the left with either a large step or hop, landing on your left leg. Hop or step back to the right.

2. As you land on one foot, cross the opposite leg a little behind you and the opposite arm in front.

3. Each time you land, make sure your knees and hips are slightly bent so you feel your thighs working and your muscles absorb the impact of the landing.

MODIFICATIONS/TIPS: **For a beginner version, step from side to side slowly to begin. Start to cross the opposite leg a little behind you and the opposite arm in front. Work on this movement pattern until you've mastered it. It will feel like light aerobics. Once you feel confident with this pattern, you can start to add a slight squat or hop.**

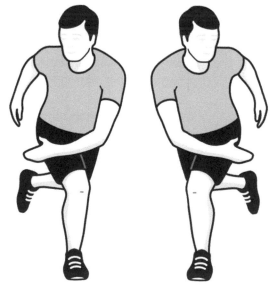

Chair Squats

MUSCLES WORKED:

▶ **Quadriceps**

▶ **Hamstrings**

▶ **Gluteus Maximus**

1. Stand a few inches in front of a chair positioned behind you, your feet hip-width apart and toes pointing straight ahead.

2. Raise both arms straight out in front of you to shoulder height. Pull your shoulder blades down and back, engaging your mid-back postural muscles.

3. Slowly sit back until your hips touch the seat of the chair. Keep your heels on the floor. Your torso will tilt forward to counterbalance the movement in your hips.

4. Hold this low position with your glutes touching the chair for a brief pause without resting in the chair.

5. Squeeze your glutes and straighten your legs back to a standing position.

MODIFICATIONS/TIPS:
Make sure your knees point in the same direction as your toes. If the knees dive in toward each other or poke out to the sides, slow down and create more tension in your inner and outer thighs to control your descent.

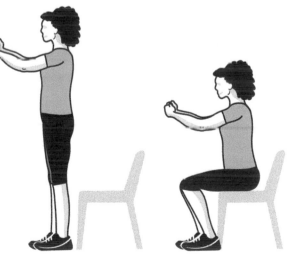

Single-Leg Chair Squat

MUSCLES WORKED:
- ▶ Quadriceps
- ▶ Hamstrings
- ▶ Gluteus Maximus

1. Stand a few inches in front of a chair positioned behind you, with your feet together.

2. Raise both arms straight out in front of you to shoulder height. Pull your shoulder blades down and back, engaging your mid-back postural muscles.

3. Balance on your right foot and engage your core muscles to raise your straight left leg off the floor at a 45-degree angle with your ankle flexed.

4. Keeping your left leg in the air, sit your hips back to touch the seat of the chair. Keep your right foot fully planted on the floor and slightly tilt your torso forward to counterbalance the movement in your hips.

5. Hold this low position with your glutes touching the chair for a brief pause before you rise and straighten your right leg back to a single-leg balance position.

6. Repeat the sequence for the desired number of repetitions, then switch to the opposite side.

MODIFICATIONS/TIPS: **If you feel unstable doing this exercise, keep the heel of your straight leg in contact with the floor to add stability and assistance.**

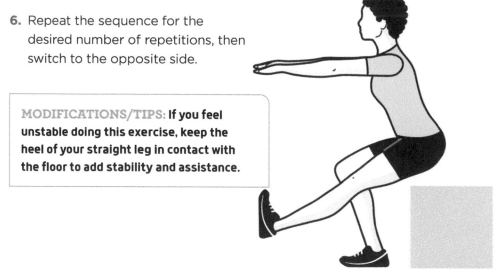

Squat

MUSCLES WORKED:
- ▶ Quadriceps
- ▶ Hamstrings
- ▶ Gluteus Maximus

1. Stand with your feet a little wider than hip-width apart and toes turned out slightly.

2. Raise both arms straight out in front of you to shoulder height. Pull your shoulder blades down and back, engaging your mid-back postural muscles.

3. Keeping your weight in your hips and heels, sit back until your thighs are parallel to the floor. Your torso will slightly tilt forward. Keep your gaze straight ahead with your chin slightly pitched down to avoid straining your neck and upper back muscles.

4. Hold this position as if you are sitting in an imaginary chair. You should feel your glutes and back squeezing to keep you from falling backward.

5. Press your feet into the floor and rise to a standing position.

6. Inhale as you lower, exhale as you rise.

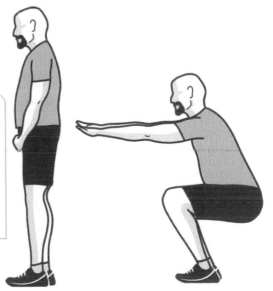

MODIFICATIONS/TIPS: **If you have trouble keeping your heels in contact with the ground on the way into the squat, try the exercise with your heels lifted on a small board (1 or 2 inches high). Keep your heels on the platform as you sit your hips back.**

Standing Side-Leg Raises

MUSCLES WORKED:
- ▶ **Glutes**
- ▶ **Quadriceps**

1. Standing straight, shift your center of gravity so you are balancing tall on your left leg.

2. Engage the thigh muscles on your right leg and raise it sideways to about 45 degrees or as high as you can lift it without rotating your hips. Flex your foot to help keep the muscles on the front and side of this leg engaged.

3. Hold for 3 seconds before slowly lowering it back down next to the left leg. You should feel this in the outer thighs on both the standing and moving legs.

4. Keep the right foot off the ground and repeat for the desired number of repetitions. Hold on to a wall or chair for balance if necessary, making sure not to lean into it. Exhale as the leg goes up, and inhale on the way down.

5. Repeat on the opposite side.

MODIFICATIONS/TIPS: **This is an entirely lateral movement with no hip, knee, or ankle rotation. Make sure your hips, knees, and ankles on both legs point straight ahead throughout the movements.**

Standing March to Crunch

MUSCLES WORKED:
▶ **Quadriceps**
▶ **Abdominals**

1. Stand with your feet together and arms straight overhead.

2. Engage your abdominal muscles to lift your right thigh parallel to the ground and bent at the knee.

3. Keep the right thigh up as you swing your arms down to clap together underneath the right thigh.

4. Lower your right leg as you simultaneously lift your arms back overhead and clap together as you would in a jumping jack.

5. Repeat with the left leg. Exhale with the under-leg clap and inhale as you lift your arms overhead.

6. If you are having difficulty with this exercise, try marching in place slowly while touching your hands to the top of the risen thigh. Hold the risen position for 3 seconds before alternating legs.

> **MODIFICATIONS/TIPS: When bending forward, engage your abdominals to avoid putting too much pressure on your lower back.**

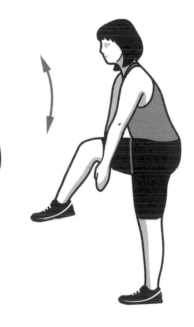

Stationary Lunge

MUSCLES WORKED:
► Quadriceps
► Hamstrings
► Gluteus Maximus
► Gastrocnemius

1. Stand in a split stance with your right foot in front and left foot behind you. Keep your legs in line with your hips. Lift your left heel off the floor. Distribute your weight between the full right foot in front and the ball of the left foot in back.

2. Bend your knees deeply and lower your body so your left knee hovers a couple of inches over the floor and your right knee comes forward directly over your right ankle. Keep your right heel on the floor and your left heel lifted while the knees are bending. You should feel a stretch or burning in the left thigh and a pull in the right hamstring and glute.

3. Push from the back of the right leg and straighten both legs, returning to starting position. Keep your torso erect and moving straight up and down like an elevator as you bend and straighten the legs.

4. Repeat the sequence for the desired number of repetitions, then switch to the opposite side.

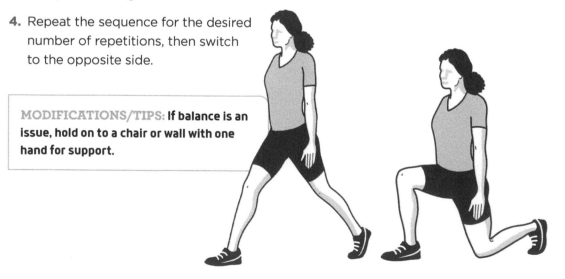

MODIFICATIONS/TIPS: **If balance is an issue, hold on to a chair or wall with one hand for support.**

Bridge

MUSCLES WORKED:
- ► **Gluteus Maximus**
- ► **Hamstrings**

1. Lie on your back with your knees bent and feet flat on the floor, legs hip-width apart. Place your arms flat on the floor right next to your body.

2. Engage your core by taking a full breath in and out, drawing in your belly button on the exhale. Push your heels firmly into the floor as you squeeze your glutes to lift your hips as high as they can go without arching your back.

3. Squeeze your glutes for another second at the top of the motion, then slowly lower all the way to the ground and gently tap the floor with your glutes before squeezing up again.

4. Keep your knees in line with your hips; not caving in or poking out.

> **MODIFICATIONS/TIPS:** You'll want to feel this movement in your glutes and hamstrings but not your lower back. Engage your lower abdominals at the start of this exercise and slightly tilt your pelvis back so your tailbone is slightly tucked under. Keep your shoulders on the floor as you lift.

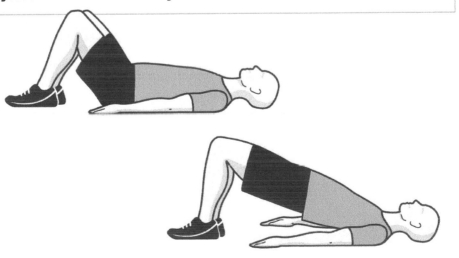

Single-Leg Bridge

MUSCLES WORKED:
- ▶ **Gluteus Maximus**
- ▶ **Hamstrings**
- ▶ **Rectus Abdominis**

1. Lie on your back with your legs together, knees bent, and feet flat on the floor. Lay your arms flat on the floor right next to your body.

2. Engage your abdominals and lift your left foot up, drawing your knee toward your chest.

3. Plant your right foot into the floor and drive up through your right heel to raise your hips and lower back as high as you can.

4. Hold for 2 seconds at the top and then control the descent as you return your hips to the floor.

5. Repeat the sequence for the desired number of repetitions, then switch to the opposite side.

> MODIFICATIONS/TIPS: **If you get a cramp during this exercise, try stretching your hamstrings first (page 32). Focus on squeezing your butt to do the bridge.**

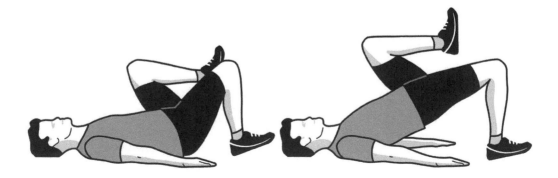

Elevated Single-Leg Bridge

MUSCLES WORKED:
- ▶ **Gluteus Maximus**
- ▶ **Hamstrings**
- ▶ **Rectus Abdominis**

1. Lean your upper back on a bench or couch, extending your arms out to the sides for support and stability.

2. With your feet together and flat on the floor, lift your hips into a high bridge so they are level with your shoulders. You should feel the effort in your glutes.

3. Lift your right foot off the floor, bringing your knee in the air.

4. Holding this leg in the air, lower your hips down toward the floor. Squeeze your glutes again to lift back up.

5. Repeat the sequence for the desired number of repetitions, then switch to the opposite side.

> MODIFICATIONS/TIPS: **This exercise is a more challenging progression from the Single-Leg Bridge (page 80). Be sure you are strong and stable in the Single-Leg Bridge before attempting this one.**

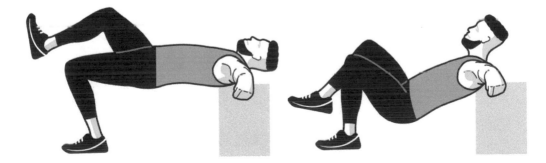

Plie Squat

MUSCLES WORKED:
▶ **Glutes**
▶ **Adductors**

1. Stand with your feet wider than hip-width apart and your toes turned out slightly.

2. Push your hips back and squat down, keeping your torso erect. Lower your knees and hips at the same speed, with your knees turned out at the same angle as your toes. Keep your heels on the floor.

3. Go as low as you can with good posture and heels on the floor. Keep tension in your thighs as you lower yourself so you don't overstretch the groin muscles.

4. Straighten your legs and push yourself back up to standing position.

MODIFICATIONS/TIPS: **If you are still building your strength to squat deeply, find something to hold on to in front of you, and let your body hang from your arms a bit as you do the exercise. This will take some weight off the legs.**

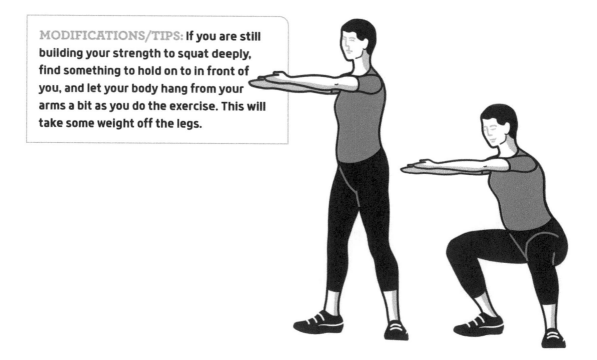

Bulgarian Lunge

MUSCLES WORKED:
- ► **Glutes**
- ► **Quadriceps**
- ► **Hamstrings**

1. Stand with a low step or chair behind you.

2. Begin in the **Stationary Lunge** starting position (see page 78) with your back leg elevated on the step. The higher the step up, the more strength and flexibility is required to perform the exercise. Keep your front toes and knee pointing straight ahead.

3. Bend both knees deeply and lower your body so the back knee hovers a couple of inches over the floor and the front knee comes forward right over the ankle. Keep your front heel grounded while the knees are bending. You will feel a stretch in the back thigh above the knee and a pull in the front leg's hamstring and glute.

4. Push through the heel of your front leg to straighten it out.

5. Repeat the sequence for the desired number of repetitions, then switch to the opposite side.

6. For a deeper stretch on the front of the body, lift your arms up overhead at the bottom of the movement.

MODIFICATIONS/TIPS: **Hold on to a chair or something sturdy for balance during step 2.**

LOWER BODY (Calves)

Toe Taps

MUSCLES WORKED:
▶ **Glutes**
▶ **Gastrocnemius**
▶ **Soleus**

1. Stand a few inches from a platform or step in front of you. The height of the step can be 12 inches or less. If you are a beginner or have tightness in your knees or hips, try a lower step.

2. Place your feet hip-width apart with arms at your sides.

3. Lift your right leg up and tap those toes on the top of the step.

4. Bring that foot back to the ground and repeat with the left foot.

5. Continue alternating this motion and add an opposite-arm pump: As your right leg lifts, pump the left arm forward as if you were jogging in place.

6. Once you feel comfortable with this movement pattern, switch back and forth with a little more speed and a small hop. You should feel the effort in your glutes and calves, and your heart rate will go up with your faster pace. Make sure you are exhaling through the switches and keeping a somewhat even tempo.

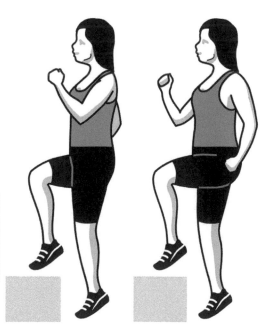

> MODIFICATIONS/TIPS: **Ensure that your step is secure and the space around the step is clear in case you lose your balance.**

Plie Squat with Heel Lift

MUSCLES WORKED:
- ▶ **Glutes**
- ▶ **Adductors**
- ▶ **Gastrocnemius**
- ▶ **Soleus**

1. Stand with your feet wider than hip-width apart and toes turned out slightly.

2. Push your hips back and squat down, keeping your torso erect. Lower your knees and hips at the same speed, with your knees turned out at the same angle as your toes. Keep your heels on the floor.

3. Go as low as you can with good posture and heels on the floor. Hold this position. If you have tight inner thighs, lower yourself slowly to protect your groin muscles from overstretching.

4. While holding the deepest position in the wide squat, lift both heels up high and balance on arched feet.

5. Lower your heels back to the floor, then straighten your legs and push yourself back up to standing position.

MODIFICATIONS/TIPS: **For an easier version, instead of lifting both heels, hold your squat at the lowest position, then lift your right heel and hold it up for 1 second, then lift the left heel and hold for 1 second before returning to stand. If you feel off-balance, hold on to a ledge in front of you.**

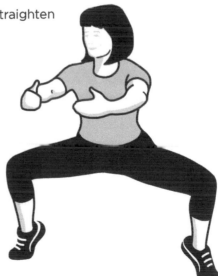

Squat to Tiptoes with Arm Swing

MUSCLES WORKED:
▶ **Glutes**
▶ **Quadriceps**
▶ **Hamstrings**
▶ **Gastrocnemius**
▶ **Soleus**

1. Stand with your feet slightly wider than hip-width apart and toes turned out slightly.

2. Lift your arms straight overhead.

3. Keeping your weight in your hips and heels, swing your arms back by your sides and sit back into a squat with your thighs parallel to the floor. Your torso will slightly tilt forward.

4. Swing your arms back overhead as you thrust your hips forward through a standing position to balance high on your tiptoes.

5. Inhale as you lower and exhale as you rise. Keep your spine in a neutral position. You should feel a stretch in the back of your hamstrings at the bottom of the movement and tightening in your glutes as you rise.

6. Balancing on your tiptoes might cause you to wobble at first. Try using your arms and legs together to give you more power getting up to your toes.

> **MODIFICATIONS/TIPS:** For a beginner version, keep your hands on your hips and perform a slow squat up to tiptoes. Once your feet are used to holding the top position for a few seconds, add the arm movement.

Heel Lift

MUSCLES WORKED:
- ▶ **Gastrocnemius**
- ▶ **Soleus**
- ▶ **Glutes**

1. Stand with your heels under your hips and your toes turned in so they are touching. Lightly hold on to something for balance.

2. Lift your heels up as high as you can and hold yourself up tall on your tiptoes. Keep the internal rotation of your thighs as you lift.

3. Slowly lower your heels down to starting position.

MODIFICATIONS/TIPS: **Try this exercise barefoot to strengthen even more muscles in your foot.**

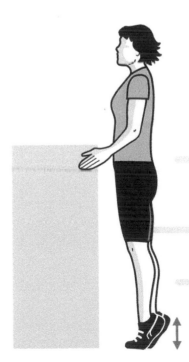

Single-Leg Heel Lift against the Wall

MUSCLES WORKED:
▶ **Gastrocnemius**

1. Stand facing a wall or ledge and hold on for balance.

2. Cross your left foot behind your right ankle so it is hooked around the leg and resting on the back of the calf.

3. Lift up as high as you can on your right toes and pause at the highest height, bringing your left foot along for the ride.

4. Lower your right heel back to the floor, taking the left foot with you.

5. Inhale on the way down and exhale on the way up.

6. Repeat the sequence for the desired number of repetitions, then switch to the opposite side.

MODIFICATIONS/TIPS: **If you spend a lot of time in high-heeled shoes or on your feet, it's essential to stretch your calves out after doing this exercise.**

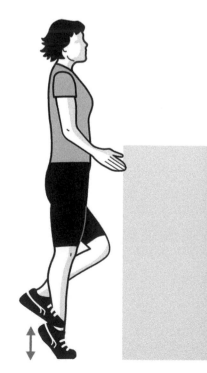

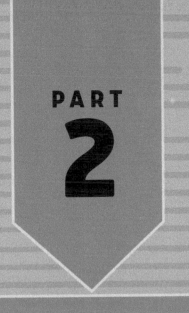

Your Bodyweight Training Routine

IN PART 2, YOU'LL FIND TWELVE WEEKS OF BODYWEIGHT workouts. Each chapter will cover three weeks corresponding to a different skill and intensity level—beginner, intermediate, advanced, and expert. For each week's workout sequence, there will be guidance on how many times you should work out, how long you should rest, and what you should do for warm-ups and cooldowns. You'll also find questions that will help you check in with yourself—how you feel, the extent of your progress, and the levels of your motivation and support.

chapter 4

BEGINNER PROGRAM

In this chapter, we will take the exercises you learned in chapter 3 and create a total bodyweight workout plan for the first three weeks of your fitness journey. You'll want to keep chapter 3 handy as a reference, especially if you have never done the exercises before. Every workout will have tips and modifications so you can personalize your program and ensure that you're exercising at a level that challenges you in a beneficial way.

WEEK ONE
beginner

Welcome to the first week of your twelve-week fitness program. Be sure to record and monitor your progress so you can keep track of where you started and how much you've improved at the end of the twelve weeks. Note how you felt before and after this week's workout.

The exercises for this first week may seem simple, but don't be surprised if you tire quickly or feel sore the next day. You're not only building a muscular foundation this week—you're also making neural connections by teaching your muscles the movement patterns that will prepare your body for optimal function in the weeks ahead.

The hardest thing about exercise
is getting started, but it won't take
long before you start to feel
the benefits. What you do this week,
your future self will thank you for!

Days of the Week: 3 times a week, with a day or two between workouts

Approximate Time: 30 to 35 minutes, with a 5-minute warm-up and 5-minute cooldown

Overview: Complete exercises 1 through 8 for one circuit, resting for 30 to 60 seconds between each exercise. Repeat for a second circuit. If you need to rest between circuits, try to keep it under 3 minutes.

Warm-Up: Easy movement to elevate your core temperature, such as brisk walking, light jogging, or aerobics

Cooldown: 4 to 5 upper- and lower-body stretches

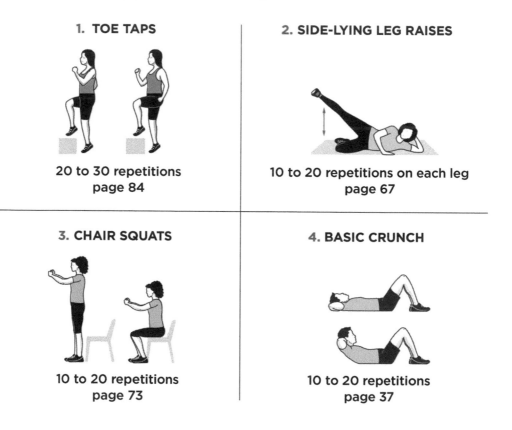

1. TOE TAPS

20 to 30 repetitions
page 84

2. SIDE-LYING LEG RAISES

10 to 20 repetitions on each leg
page 67

3. CHAIR SQUATS

10 to 20 repetitions
page 73

4. BASIC CRUNCH

10 to 20 repetitions
page 37

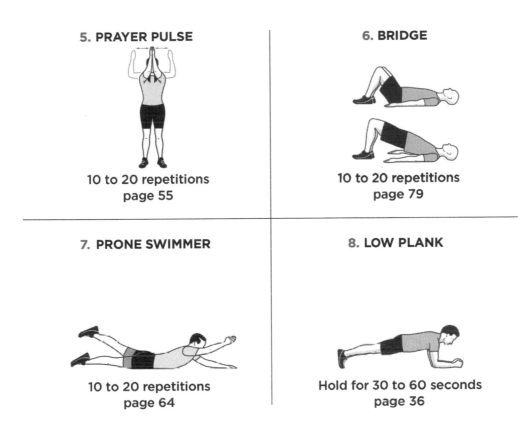

5. PRAYER PULSE

10 to 20 repetitions
page 55

6. BRIDGE

10 to 20 repetitions
page 79

7. PRONE SWIMMER

10 to 20 repetitions
page 64

8. LOW PLANK

Hold for 30 to 60 seconds
page 36

MODIFICATIONS The order of exercises in this week's program enlists the peripheral heart action training modality (see page 19) and alternates between standing and floor exercises for greater cardiovascular benefit. If you find that getting up and down frequently is too strenuous or makes you dizzy, do all the odd-numbered exercises in a row and then the even-numbered ones—this way you'll be standing for the first half of the circuit and on the floor for the second half.

TO YOUR LEVEL

This first week, you are laying the foundation to build a stronger body. All this week's exercises are basic, but not necessarily easy. If you're new to bodyweight training, complete one circuit instead of two for the first week, as you are building stamina. If after completing the first circuit you are looking for a greater challenge, shorten your rest time between exercises or add a third set.

Self Check-In

1. **Am I energized or fatigued after my workouts?**

   » *Sleep is a big factor in your body's readiness to exercise and ability to recover. Now's a great time to make sure you're getting enough sleep.*

2. **Did I feel confident I was doing the exercises in the correct form?**

   » *Read over the instructions before starting your workout, and keep your exercise guide handy so you can refer back to it as needed.*

3. **Did my appetite increase, and did I refuel with healthy carbs, fat, and protein?**

   » *When you first start a workout program, sometimes you will feel hungry for a day after your workout. Respond to this hunger with foods that fuel you, rather than with junk food and sugar. Try eating more protein, especially at night, to feel more satiated.*

4. **Do I have a support system to share my progress with?**

   » *Start telling your friends and loved ones that you're making positive changes to your lifestyle. Their support will help you stay motivated and accountable.*

WEEK TWO
beginner

This week, you'll be working on a whole new set of exercises, continuing to build your foundation. These exercises are slightly more dynamic and involve more compound movements. As you start this week, keep monitoring your progress by recording your workouts and how you're feeling. Write down your triumphs as well as your struggles. Be proud of your success and that you've stayed committed to a healthier lifestyle. If you encounter some areas of difficulty this week, make a note so you can pay more attention to areas for improvement.

The bank of your body has the best interest rate you can find.
Think of each workout as a deposit that will pay you back in longevity, vitality, and years of good health.

Days of the Week: 3 times a week, with a day or two between workouts

Approximate Time: 30 to 35 minutes, with 5-minute warm-up and 5-minute cooldown

Overview: Complete exercises 1 through 8 for one circuit, resting for 30 to 60 seconds between each exercise. Repeat for a second circuit. If you need to rest between circuits, try to keep it under 3 minutes.

Warm-Up: Easy movement to elevate your core temperature, such as brisk walking, light jogging, or aerobics

Cooldown: 4 to 5 upper- and lower-body stretches

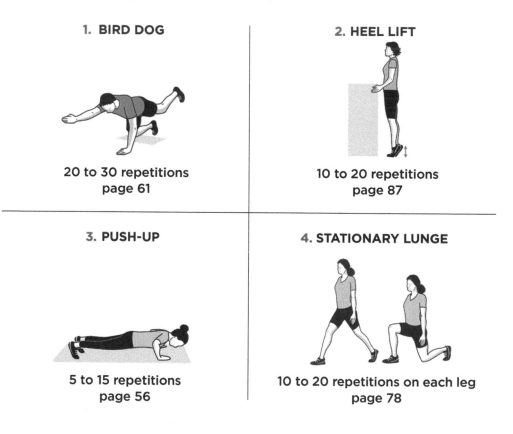

1. BIRD DOG

20 to 30 repetitions
page 61

2. HEEL LIFT

10 to 20 repetitions
page 87

3. PUSH-UP

5 to 15 repetitions
page 56

4. STATIONARY LUNGE

10 to 20 repetitions on each leg
page 78

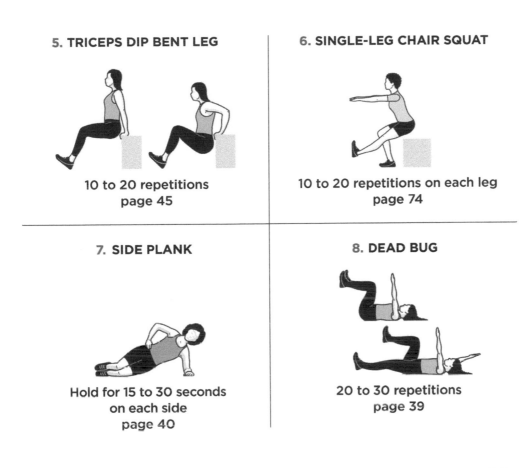

5. TRICEPS DIP BENT LEG

10 to 20 repetitions
page 45

6. SINGLE-LEG CHAIR SQUAT

10 to 20 repetitions on each leg
page 74

7. SIDE PLANK

Hold for 15 to 30 seconds
on each side
page 40

8. DEAD BUG

20 to 30 repetitions
page 39

MODIFICATIONS There is a lot of focus on shoulders and calves in this week's workout. If your shoulders or lower legs get fatigued easily, maybe from past injury, give yourself a slow and gentle counter-stretch immediately after the exercise you find strenuous. For example, after **Triceps Dip Bent Leg**, spend 30 seconds doing **Wall Stretch for Chest** (page 26); after doing **Stationary Lunge**, spend 30 seconds doing each side of **Standing Calf Stretch** (page 30) and **Standing Quadriceps Stretch** (page 31).

TO YOUR LEVEL

Your body is likely more prepared this week for the length of the workout, but if you find stamina to be a challenge, it's okay to take longer rests between exercises. The **Push-Up**, **Stationary Lunge**, and **Side Plank** are the most complex in this set, so give yourself some time to set up properly and check your form. Check each exercise's instructions in chapter 3 for suggestions on how to make things easier. If you want a bigger challenge for this week's suggested circuit, slow down the exercises to extend the time each muscle stays engaged. You can also shorten your rest time between exercises or add a third set.

Self Check-In

1. **How challenging was my workout?**
   » *Workouts should always have a level of challenge, but it shouldn't be so hard that you feel like you can't finish or you dread coming back. If you find the workout daunting, use the easier modifications suggested for each exercise and stick with a low-repetition range until you have more confidence. Consider going through them with a personal trainer or friend who is experienced with working out.*

2. **Were you as motivated to exercise this week as last week?**
   » *Check in with your support system and let them be your cheerleading squad. Take some time to reflect on why you started, and keep it in mind. Revisit your goal worksheet (page 9).*

3. **Are you drinking at least eight glasses of water a day?**
   » *It's important to stay hydrated. Hydration supports all systems in the body to do their best work.*

4. **How sore are you after every workout?**
   » *It's good to be mildly sore after most workouts, but if you are feeling debilitated by soreness the day after every workout, you might be working too hard.*

WEEK THREE
beginner

This is your final week of "foundation-building" workouts. These first three weeks of workouts are designed to provide both a challenge and a feeling of accomplishment. If, by the end of this week, you are feeling unsteady or out of control in your body, it can help to return to the exercises in week 1 and keep working on building your foundation. Muscle soreness is also expected to a degree after most workouts, but if you're finding every workout is still leaving you hobbling up and down stairs the next day, you may want to return to week 1. Be assured, you're still making progress, but everyone progresses differently, and if you aren't quite ready to move on to the next chapter, you'll still be getting all the healthy fitness benefits by circling back to weeks 1 through 3.

Your body is a powerful force of strength, resilience, and perseverance. You have the power within you to get fit and stay fit.

Days of the Week: 3 times a week, with a day or two between workouts

Approximate Time: 30 to 35 minutes, with 10-minute warm-up and 5-minute cooldown

Overview: Complete exercises 1 through 8 for one circuit, resting for 30 to 60 seconds between each exercise. Repeat for a second circuit. If you need to rest between circuits, try to keep it under 3 minutes.

Warm-Up: Easy movement to elevate your core temperature, such as brisk walking, light jogging, or aerobics. Complete the first 5 minutes at the same intensity as week 1 and 2, and for the next 5 minutes, increase your intensity to a more vigorous level.

Cooldown: 4 to 5 upper- and lower-body stretches

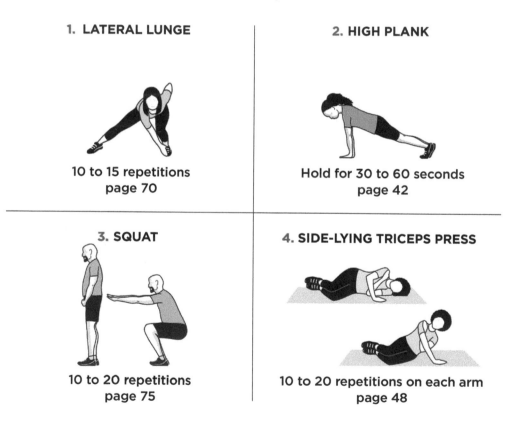

1. LATERAL LUNGE

10 to 15 repetitions
page 70

2. HIGH PLANK

Hold for 30 to 60 seconds
page 42

3. SQUAT

10 to 20 repetitions
page 75

4. SIDE-LYING TRICEPS PRESS

10 to 20 repetitions on each arm
page 48

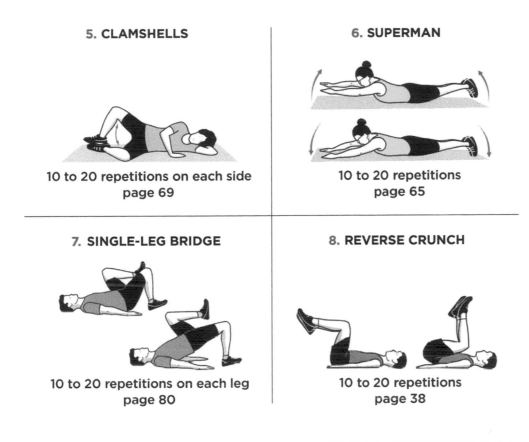

5. CLAMSHELLS

10 to 20 repetitions on each side
page 69

6. SUPERMAN

10 to 20 repetitions
page 65

7. SINGLE-LEG BRIDGE

10 to 20 repetitions on each leg
page 80

8. REVERSE CRUNCH

10 to 20 repetitions
page 38

MODIFICATIONS If you have a history of back injury, you may want to modify or replace the **Superman** exercise or the **Single-Leg Bridge**. If you feel achy in your lower back when trying these exercises, replace **Superman** with the **Prone Swimmer** (page 64) and the **Single-Leg Bridge** with the **Bridge** (page 79) until you feel stronger in your glutes and core.

TO YOUR LEVEL

It's always important to focus on form, but you'll really want to do this group of exercises with precision and focus your mind on the targeted muscle. If you find these exercises simple and want a greater challenge, you can slow down your reps and maintain control through the higher end of the repetition range. If this circuit feels too advanced, it's fine to stick with the lower number of repetitions and just focus on keeping a smooth, even tempo—not too fast, not too slow. As always, don't forget to breathe!

Self Check-In

1. **Have I been getting very out of breath during the workout?**

   » *In addition to your bodyweight training workouts, you could add one or two days a week of light cardio on your rest days to increase your lung capacity.*

2. **Am I keeping a record of my workouts?**

   » *It can be encouraging to see how you have progressed since you started!*

3. **Am I eating healthy meals that provide good nutrition?**

   » *Pairing your workout with healthy eating habits will help you feel stronger and see the best results from all your hard work.*

4. **Did I exercise with as much intensity as I could have?**

   » *Now that you've established exercise as a regular part of your life, you can start to push yourself a little outside your comfort zone for even better results.*

Beginner Program Notes

Use these pages to take down notes for each week of your workout. Reflect on your strengths and weaknesses. Do you have favorite exercises? Exercises that need some extra work? Did you notice any trends on days you felt particularly good? Did certain meals affect your workouts?

WEEK ONE

WEEK TWO

WEEK THREE

INTERMEDIATE PROGRAM

Congratulations! You've graduated to the next level of workouts. In the first three weeks of workouts, you built muscular strength to advance your bodyweight training and incorporated exercises that require greater core strength and coordination. We talked a lot in chapter 4 about building your foundation. Now that you have a solid foundation in bodyweight training, the real fun can begin.

WEEK ONE
intermediate

As your workouts become more dynamic this week, remember to stay hydrated throughout the day and replenish yourself with nourishing food—this puts you in the best place to recover quickly and feel good while you're working out. Also this week, the movements get more complex, which means you'll need to focus on form even more. Take your time and make sure you have control over the movements. If you are able to complete the workout three times this week, by the third workout day you should be able to speed things up a bit, but listen to your body—everyone progresses differently.

Whenever you exercise,
you are making positive changes
to your muscles, heart,
and mind. Let yourself be proud
of how far you've come.

Days of the Week: 3 times a week, with a day or two between workouts

Approximate Time: 30 to 35 minutes, with 5-minute warm-up and 5-minute cooldown

Overview: This week's workout is broken up into two circuits of 4 exercises each. Complete exercises 1 through 4 to complete one circuit, and then repeat for a second circuit. Rest no more than 3 minutes between each circuit. Then complete exercises 5 through 8 for one circuit and repeat for a second circuit. Rest for 30 to 60 seconds between each exercise.

Warm-Up: Moderate-intensity movement to elevate your core temperature, such as brisk walking, light jogging, aerobics, stairs, or cycling

Cooldown: 4 to 5 upper- and lower-body stretches

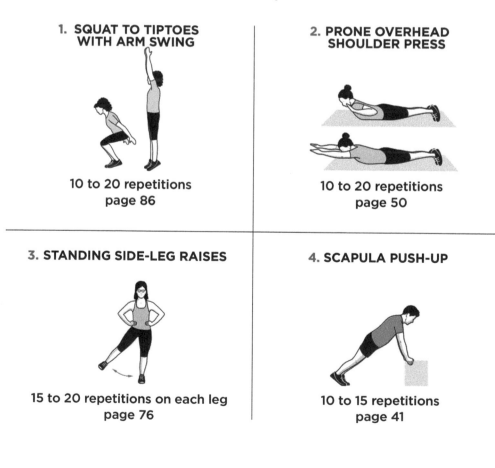

1. SQUAT TO TIPTOES WITH ARM SWING

10 to 20 repetitions
page 86

2. PRONE OVERHEAD SHOULDER PRESS

10 to 20 repetitions
page 50

3. STANDING SIDE-LEG RAISES

15 to 20 repetitions on each leg
page 76

4. SCAPULA PUSH-UP

10 to 15 repetitions
page 41

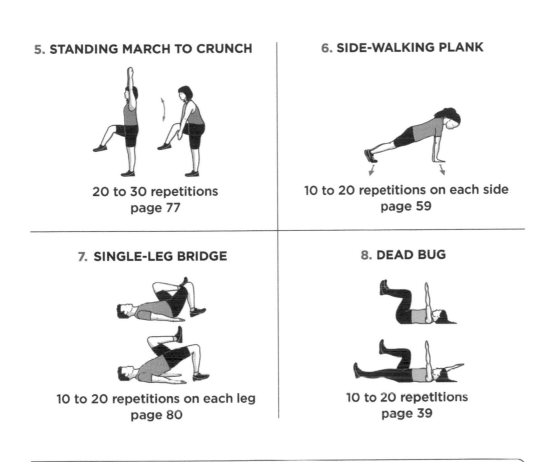

5. STANDING MARCH TO CRUNCH

20 to 30 repetitions
page 77

6. SIDE-WALKING PLANK

10 to 20 repetitions on each side
page 59

7. SINGLE-LEG BRIDGE

10 to 20 repetitions on each leg
page 80

8. DEAD BUG

10 to 20 repetitions
page 39

MODIFICATIONS You'll find some greater core challenges in this week's workout, so make sure you are feeling strong and able to hold a **High Plank** (page 42) and **Low Plank** (page 36) confidently for more than 30 seconds before attempting the **Side-Walking Plank** and **Scapula Push-Up**.

TO YOUR LEVEL

Even if you finished strong on week 3 in the Beginner Level and were doing the higher end of the repetition range, you don't have to start there for this week. These new exercises use more body parts, which will increase your cardiovascular effort, so if you want to start with the lower recommended repetitions the first time you do the workout, you can always increase reps as you gain confidence over the course of the week. Conversely, if you want a greater challenge, go for the higher end of the repetition range and rest only 30 seconds or so between exercises.

Self Check-In

1. **Am I having fun?**

   » *Try putting some of your favorite music on in the background while you're exercising.*

2. **Am I taking care of myself by getting seven to eight hours of sleep a night and drinking eight or more glasses of water a day?**

   » *You'll have much more energy for your workouts and other parts of your life if you are well rested and hydrated.*

3. **Am I celebrating my success?**

   » *Share your accomplishments with your support system—especially those who are really cheering you on. Reward yourself, too, especially after a good workout or on your rest days, such as with a favorite activity or just a long shower.*

4. **Have I noticed the strength benefits of my bodyweight training program in any other areas of my life?**

   » *Once you start realizing those stairs you climb at the office are a little easier, or you're actually keeping up with your grandkids while they're running around, you'll feel like you always want to keep fitness in your life.*

WEEK TWO
intermediate

Your body should be accustomed to regular exercise now and will thrive this week while revisiting some old favorites from chapter 4. You'll also be combining aspects of foundational exercises like a **Push-Up** (page 56) with a **Side Plank** (page 40), stimulating new muscular growth and adaptation.

You have found the true
fountain of youth—
regular exercise. Think
of it as your free
anti-aging supplement.

Days of the Week: 3 times a week, with a day or two between workouts

Approximate Time: 30 to 35 minutes, with 5-minute warm-up and 5-minute cooldown

Overview: Complete exercises 1 through 4 to complete one circuit and then repeat for a second circuit. Rest no more than 3 minutes between each circuit. Then complete exercises 5 through 8 for one circuit and then repeat for a second circuit. Rest for 30 to 60 seconds between each exercise.

Warm-Up: Moderate-intensity movement to elevate your core temperature, such as brisk walking, light jogging, aerobics, stairs, or cycling

Cooldown: 4 to 5 upper- and lower-body stretches

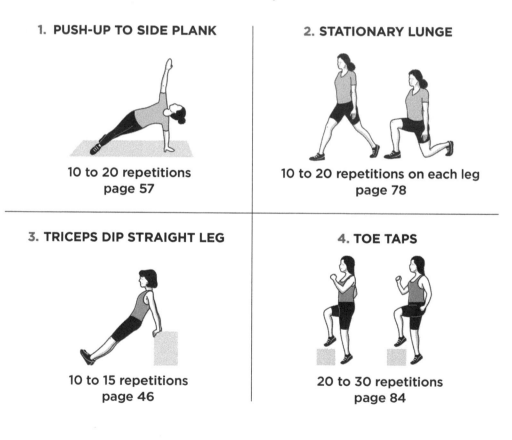

1. PUSH-UP TO SIDE PLANK

10 to 20 repetitions
page 57

2. STATIONARY LUNGE

10 to 20 repetitions on each leg
page 78

3. TRICEPS DIP STRAIGHT LEG

10 to 15 repetitions
page 46

4. TOE TAPS

20 to 30 repetitions
page 84

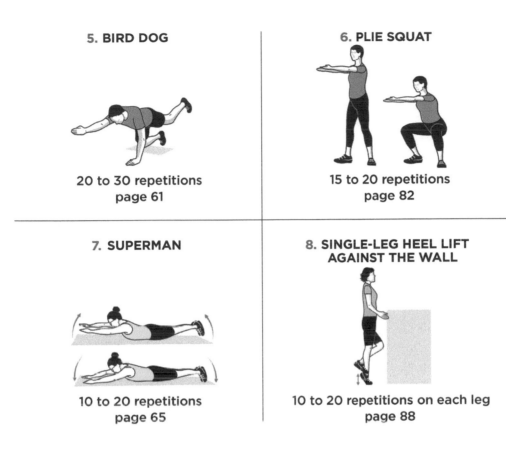

5. BIRD DOG

20 to 30 repetitions
page 61

6. PLIE SQUAT

15 to 20 repetitions
page 82

7. SUPERMAN

10 to 20 repetitions
page 65

**8. SINGLE-LEG HEEL LIFT
AGAINST THE WALL**

10 to 20 repetitions on each leg
page 88

MODIFICATIONS Pay close attention to your breath and form on the combined movements in this workout. **Push-Up to Side Plank**, **Stationary Lunge**, **Triceps Dip Straight Leg**, and **Plie Squat** engage more muscles at the same time than some other exercises, so take your time and start with the lower repetition range if you need to. The quality of your exercise is more important than quantity in producing desired results.

TO YOUR LEVEL

This week's workout is broken up into two circuits of four exercises each. Try doing exercises 1 through 4 for two circuits and then exercises 5 through 8 for two circuits. For a beginner approach, do the two circuits for two sets each and keep the repetition range on the lower end. Repetition is important for strength building and forming neurological connections in your muscles, so doing that second set will have great benefits. If you want a greater challenge, do all eight exercises in a row for a third circuit after you've completed the other two rounds.

Self Check-In

1. **Are you more flexible than when you started working out five weeks ago?**
    » *Maybe you can touch your toes more easily or reach a high cabinet. If not, spend a little more time on the stretches after your workouts.*

2. **Have your mood and attitude improved since you started exercising?**
    » *Exercise produces endorphins, which make you feel good, and over time, it increases dopamine levels, which improves your mood and attitude.*

3. **Do you think about breathing during your workouts?**
    » *Your workouts will be higher quality if you consciously practice steady breathing with each movement.*

4. **Do you have enough energy to finish your workout and then remain active throughout the day?**
    » *If you aren't sustaining your energy, make sure you're getting good nutrition daily and consider looking into appropriate supplements.*

WEEK THREE
intermediate

This week's workout is full of compound movements and alternates upper- and lower-body work. It's a challenging progression of all the basics; it's also a circuit you'll want to master before moving on to the advanced programs in the next chapter. Celebrate how far you've come by having fun in this week's workouts. As always, don't forget to breathe and look out for good form.

You are stronger than you think.
When the going gets tough,
bring to mind all the people
who care about you and
are inspired by your success.

Days of the Week: 3 times a week, with a day or two between workouts

Approximate Time: 30 to 35 minutes, with 5-minute warm-up and 5-minute cooldown

Overview: Complete exercises 1 through 4 to complete one circuit and then repeat for a second circuit. Rest no more than 3 minutes between each circuit. Then complete exercises 5 through 8 for one circuit and then repeat for a second circuit. Rest for 30 to 60 seconds between each exercise.

Warm-Up: Moderate-intensity movement to elevate your core temperature, such as brisk walking, light jogging, aerobics, stairs, or cycling

Cooldown: 4 to 5 upper- and lower-body stretches

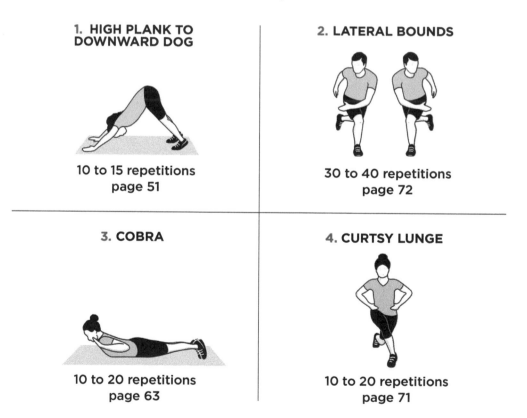

1. HIGH PLANK TO DOWNWARD DOG	2. LATERAL BOUNDS
10 to 15 repetitions page 51	30 to 40 repetitions page 72
3. COBRA	4. CURTSY LUNGE
10 to 20 repetitions page 63	10 to 20 repetitions page 71

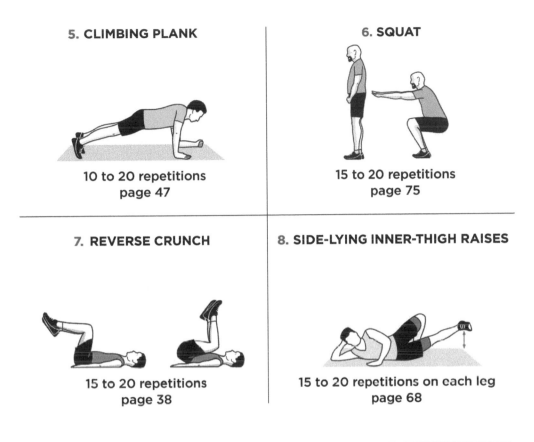

5. CLIMBING PLANK

10 to 20 repetitions
page 47

6. SQUAT

15 to 20 repetitions
page 75

7. REVERSE CRUNCH

15 to 20 repetitions
page 38

8. SIDE-LYING INNER-THIGH RAISES

15 to 20 repetitions on each leg
page 68

MODIFICATIONS These two circuits are likely to elevate your heart rate more than in previous weeks. Focus on exhaling long and slow through the hard part of the exercise, and inhale through your nose. As you get fatigued, pay close attention to posture and make sure your spine isn't slumping. Keep the tension out of your neck and shoulders by rolling your shoulders back and keeping your shoulder blades close to your middle spine.

TO YOUR LEVEL

If you are skillful at the exercises in these two circuits, do the first set at a faster tempo (without rushing) and the second set at a much slower tempo, especially during the part of the exercise where you are going in the same direction as gravity. If you have more time and energy to spare after doing both circuits for two sets, start at the beginning and do a third set of all eight exercises in a row once.

Self Check-In

1. **Have I been able to stay consistent with my workouts?**
   » *Make this appointment with yourself as important as any work meeting. Put it in your calendar.*

2. **Am I seeing changes in my body from all my hard work?**
   » *It can be motivating and confidence-boosting when you notice your new and better posture, muscle definition, and energy levels.*

3. **Do I feel more energetic and confident than I did six weeks ago?**
   » *I hope you do! If not, try to pinpoint what's missing. Is your exercise schedule regular? Are you getting enough rest, nutrition, and sleep? Is an injury or illness setting you back? Any regular exercise is progress. Try to move to your ability, and seek medical attention if challenges persist.*

4. **Am I still paying attention to hydration, sleep, and nutrition?**
   » *Keeping these components of your health in mind is essential, especially as you progress with more challenging workouts ahead.*

Intermediate Program Notes

Use these pages to take down notes for each week of your workout. Reflect on your strengths and weaknesses. Do you have favorite exercises? Exercises that need some extra work? Did you notice any trends on days you felt particularly good? Did certain meals affect your workouts?

WEEK ONE

WEEK TWO

WEEK THREE

ADVANCED PROGRAM

Your hard work and dedication have paid off, and you are officially ready for advanced bodyweight training workouts! You will have already mastered about half of the exercises in this chapter in the first six weeks of your bodyweight training program, but you'll find some new ones that require a higher level of strength, skill, and energy. I recommended approaching these challenges like a beginner. Give yourself space to reduce the repetitions and focus on form. Even though you are advanced, there might be days your body needs more rest. On those days, have patience and find a way to take it down a notch. Likewise, on the days when you are feeling strong, flaunt it like the rock star you are!

WEEK ONE
advanced

In week 1 of advanced programs, you'll find more lower-body exercises than upper-body exercises. While your legs are working hard and being challenged with endurance, take the opportunity to really focus on your form in the upper-body and core exercises since your arms won't be as tired throughout the circuit.

You'll be primarily on your feet and working the larger muscles of the legs, so you may feel more out of breath than usual. This is normal. Just remember to prioritize form and depth of movement over speed. Quality is always better than quantity to get the best results from this workout sequence. Be sure to record your workouts so you can monitor your progress.

You don't have to be perfect to make progress. Just keep showing up and doing the work—you are already transforming.

Days of the Week: 3 times a week, with a day or two between workouts

Approximate Time: 30 to 35 minutes, with 5-minute warm-up and 5-minute cooldown

Overview: Complete exercises 1 through 8 for one circuit, resting for 30 to 60 seconds between each exercise. Repeat for a second circuit after resting for no more than 3 minutes.

Warm-Up: Moderate-intensity movement to elevate your core temperature, such as brisk walking, light jogging, aerobics, stairs, or cycling. If time allows, spend an additional 5 minutes increasing your intensity to a more vigorous level.

Cooldown: 4 to 5 upper- and lower-body stretches

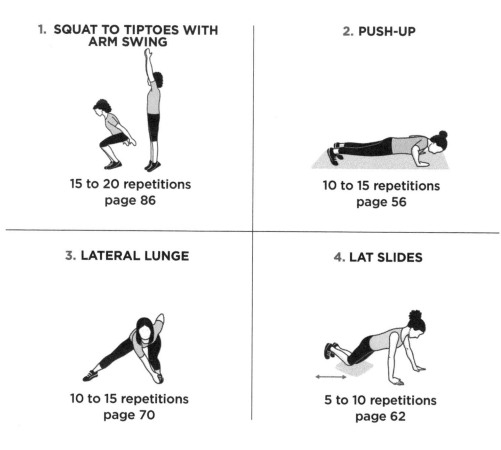

1. SQUAT TO TIPTOES WITH ARM SWING	2. PUSH-UP
15 to 20 repetitions page 86	10 to 15 repetitions page 56
3. LATERAL LUNGE	4. LAT SLIDES
10 to 15 repetitions page 70	5 to 10 repetitions page 62

5. STATIONARY LUNGE

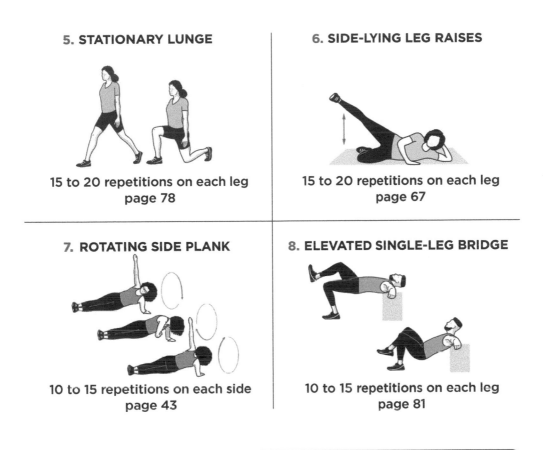

15 to 20 repetitions on each leg
page 78

6. SIDE-LYING LEG RAISES

15 to 20 repetitions on each leg
page 67

7. ROTATING SIDE PLANK

10 to 15 repetitions on each side
page 43

8. ELEVATED SINGLE-LEG BRIDGE

10 to 15 repetitions on each leg
page 81

MODIFICATIONS As mentioned, there are fewer upper-body exercises in this circuit but you can still add focus on your arms. If you are able to perform the upper repetition range on your first set, try adding an extra five to ten repetitions to the second set of **Push-Ups** and **Lat Slides**.

TO YOUR LEVEL

Push-Ups can be done on your knees, but you can also try them on your toes for more of a challenge. Even if you start the set of fifteen repetitions with only five **Push-Ups** on your toes and then complete the set on your knees, this will help you build more strength. Each time you approach the workout this week, try to complete one more repetition on your toes.

Self Check-In

1. **Am I still getting support and encouragement from my friends and family?**

   » *Surround yourself with at least a small group of people who are cheering you on. But remember your greatest cheerleader: you!*

2. **Am I taking time to plan and prepare healthy, nutritious meals?**

   » *It's important to support these advanced programs with good nutrition. If possible, plan your grocery shopping to keep your home properly stocked so you can continue making good food choices during busy weeks.*

3. **Does your body feel unbalanced or muscularly tense when you are not exercising?**

   » *Get yourself a massage or try some self-myofascial release techniques to knead the knots out of your hard-working muscles. See Resources (page 164) for a helpful link to learn more.*

4. **Aside from appropriate muscle soreness after a workout, am I feeling fatigued or worn out?**

   » *Try turning off electronic screens early at night to get restorative and restful sleep.*

WEEK TWO
advanced

Three new exercises are being incorporated into your workout this week: **Eccentric Push-Up to Cobra** (page 58), **Inverted Scapula Press-Up** (page 52), and **Bulgarian Lunge** (page 83). Your body is amply prepared to approach all of these with skill and strength, but even so, pace yourself and pay close attention to form. Once again, you'll find yourself on your feet and in positions that require the use of more body parts at once. This means both your musculoskeletal system and your cardiovascular system will be challenged throughout the program. As always, don't forget to breathe.

Fitness is just the beginning.
As you get stronger,
every aspect of your life
has the potential to thrive.

Days of the Week: 3 times a week, with a day or two between workouts

Approximate Time: 30 to 35 minutes, with 5-minute warm-up and 5-minute cooldown

Overview: Complete exercises 1 through 8 for one circuit, resting for 30 to 60 seconds between each exercise. Repeat for a second circuit after resting for no more than 3 minutes.

Warm-Up: Moderate-intensity movement to elevate your core temperature, such as brisk walking, light jogging, aerobics, stairs, or cycling. If time allows, spend an additional 5 minutes increasing your intensity to a more vigorous level.

Cooldown: 4 to 5 upper- and lower-body stretches

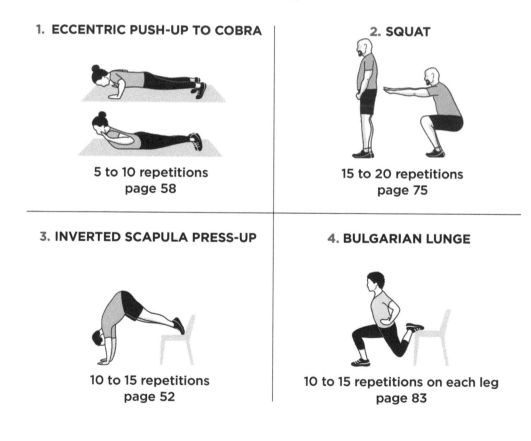

1. ECCENTRIC PUSH-UP TO COBRA

5 to 10 repetitions
page 58

2. SQUAT

15 to 20 repetitions
page 75

3. INVERTED SCAPULA PRESS-UP

10 to 15 repetitions
page 52

4. BULGARIAN LUNGE

10 to 15 repetitions on each leg
page 83

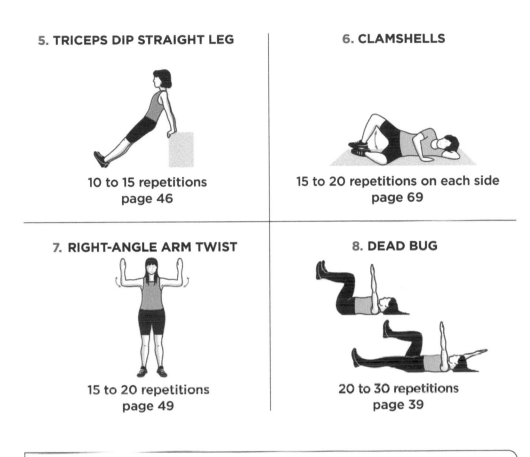

5. TRICEPS DIP STRAIGHT LEG

10 to 15 repetitions
page 46

6. CLAMSHELLS

15 to 20 repetitions on each side
page 69

7. RIGHT-ANGLE ARM TWIST

15 to 20 repetitions
page 49

8. DEAD BUG

20 to 30 repetitions
page 39

MODIFICATIONS The **Inverted Scapula Press-Up** puts your head in an upside-down position. For some, this position may cause dizziness or general discomfort. If you want to replace this with another exercise, you can use **Scapula Push-Up** (page 41) or **Prone Overhead Shoulder Press** (page 50).

TO YOUR LEVEL

This more advanced program should challenge all levels. However, if you're looking to go even deeper into your workout, start to add deep core breathing to your exercises. On the "easier" movement phase of the exercise, inhale slowly through your nose and fill your belly up with air. On the "harder" phase of the exercise (usually the part where you are working against gravity), exhale through your mouth, pushing all the air out of your belly so you feel your abdominal muscles contract deeply as you complete the movement.

Self Check-In

1. **Do I look forward to my workouts?**
   » *On those days when it's hard to get started, remember how good you feel when you're done.*

2. **Am I staying hydrated by drinking eight glasses of water throughout the day?**
   » *On days when you consume alcohol or caffeine or sweat more than usual (including hot and humid days), you may need to drink more than eight glasses to replenish yourself.*

3. **Do I have enough time to complete my workouts?**
   » *Sometimes it's hard to fit everything in, but even a short workout is better than none. If you have a very busy week, just try doing one set of everything a little faster and with more intensity. You'll still get a lot of benefit.*

4. **Do I have enough energy during and after my workouts?**
   » *If energy is an issue, make sure you're getting enough protein in your diet.*

WEEK THREE
advanced

As you move into your third week of advanced programs, you'll incorporate just a few new exercises from chapter 3. At the end of this week, you will have experienced all the bodyweight exercises recommended in this book, making this a good time to check in on your body awareness and understanding of form. If you've been diligent about recording your workouts, go back and see how far you've come and how many different movements you've put your body through. You will see your progression from simple single-joint exercises into much more complex compound movements, working more muscles more efficiently. If you're confident that your form is correct, have some fun as you advance to the next level!

Progress isn't a straight line up; it's a gradual incline. Sometimes you'll hit a bump in the road and feel like you're declining. We all have those days. Just remember, any movement is progress. Look at your results over a longer period—you'll see your progress line has been going up all along.

Days of the Week: 3 times a week, with a day or two between workouts

Approximate Time: 30 to 35 minutes, with 5-minute warm-up and 5-minute cooldown

Overview: Complete exercises 1 through 8 for one circuit, resting for 30 to 60 seconds between each exercise. Repeat for a second circuit after resting for no more than 3 minutes.

Warm-Up: Moderate-intensity movement to elevate your core temperature, such as brisk walking, light jogging, aerobics, stairs, or cycling. If time allows, spend an additional 5 minutes increasing your intensity to a more vigorous level.

Cooldown: 4 to 5 upper- and lower-body stretches

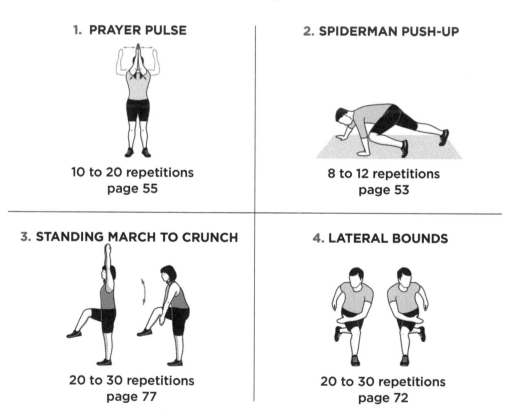

1. PRAYER PULSE

10 to 20 repetitions
page 55

2. SPIDERMAN PUSH-UP

8 to 12 repetitions
page 53

3. STANDING MARCH TO CRUNCH

20 to 30 repetitions
page 77

4. LATERAL BOUNDS

20 to 30 repetitions
page 72

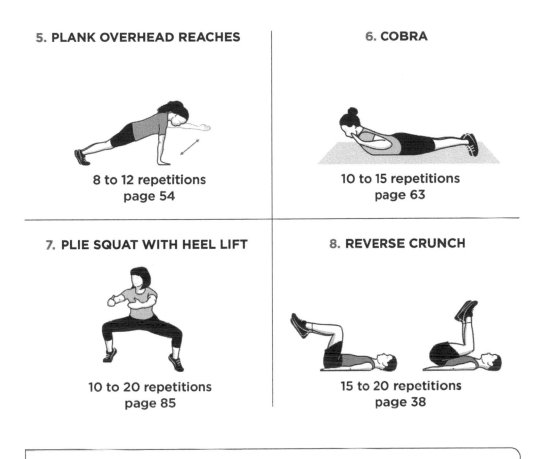

5. PLANK OVERHEAD REACHES

8 to 12 repetitions
page 54

6. COBRA

10 to 15 repetitions
page 63

7. PLIE SQUAT WITH HEEL LIFT

10 to 20 repetitions
page 85

8. REVERSE CRUNCH

15 to 20 repetitions
page 38

MODIFICATIONS It always comes back to form, breath, and core engagement. These three things are essential to get the most benefit from all your week 3 exercises. Slow things down when you are doing **Spiderman Push-Up**, **Plank Overhead Reaches**, and **Reverse Crunch**. Because these all target the core and require advanced breath work, it's important to take your time here.

TO YOUR LEVEL

If you want this circuit to offer an even greater metabolic boost (calorie burn), try adding an extra set of **Lateral Bounds** between and after the circuits. **Lateral Bounds** can remain low-impact by making the motion more of a step-cross, or higher-impact by turning your step into more of a jump. If your body is ready for a high-impact move, jumping can result in great benefits to bone density and muscular power.

Self Check-In

1. **Am I feeling and seeing results from my workouts?**
   » *After nine weeks of working out, your body should be feeling stronger and more energetic. You should have better posture and be able to see some muscle tone, especially on leaner parts of your body.*

2. **Am I spending enough time on my flexibility?**
   » *It's easy to get caught up in the workout and forget to stretch after. Stretching will help with muscle soreness, recovery, and flexibility.*

3. **How do I know if my health has improved?**
   » *One fun and easy way to see if you have gotten fitter is to measure your resting heart rate. Average resting heart rate is between sixty and eighty beats per minute—generally, the lower yours is, the fitter you are. Start measuring your resting heart rate in the morning and adding it to your workout log.*

4. **Am I working out with enough intensity?**
   » *A workout can be made more intense and effective just by changing your mindset. On days when you are feeling good, push yourself to do at least one more rep than you think you can.*

Advanced Program Notes

Use these pages to take down notes for each week of your workout. Reflect on your strengths and weaknesses. Do you have favorite exercises? Exercises that need some extra work? Did you notice any trends on days you felt particularly good? Did certain meals affect your workouts?

WEEK ONE

WEEK TWO

WEEK THREE

EXPERT PROGRAM

Welcome to chapter 7 and your expert bodyweight training program. You've done a lot of hard work to get this far and you should be incredibly proud of yourself. At this level of fitness, you'll want to find ways to have fun with your workouts so you're inspired to continue using them after you complete week 12. Consistency is the key to positive physical change when it comes to exercise, so not every workout that you finish needs to take you to the next level. Sometimes it's okay just to move your body and keep it engaged. This chapter combines even more of the complex movements from your advanced programs, but also includes some foundational exercises that are always good to return to with a deeper focus on breath and core engagement.

WEEK ONE
expert

Welcome to week 10. You're an expert now! This week's circuit combines many of the more challenging exercises in the book and should be done with a higher level of intensity. You won't see any new exercises for the next three weeks, so everything will be familiar. In the exercises you have mastered, follow the recommended modifications to take them to a higher level.

An aging body is a gift that some people never get to experience. Celebrate and honor it with daily movement. It's your birthright to discover what it's capable of.

Days of the Week: 3 times a week, with a day or two between workouts

Approximate Time: 30 to 35 minutes, with 5-minute warm-up and 5-minute cooldown

Overview: Complete exercises 1 through 4 to complete one circuit and then repeat for a second circuit. Rest no more than 3 minutes between each circuit. Then complete exercises 5 through 8 for one circuit and then repeat for a second circuit. Rest for 30 to 60 seconds between each exercise.

Warm-Up: Moderate-intensity movement to elevate your core temperature, such as brisk walking, light jogging, aerobics, stairs, or cycling. If time allows, spend an additional 5 minutes increasing your intensity to a more vigorous level.

Cooldown: 4 to 5 upper- and lower-body stretches

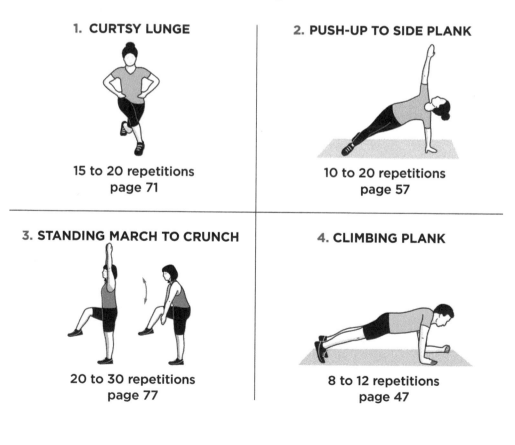

1. CURTSY LUNGE

15 to 20 repetitions
page 71

2. PUSH-UP TO SIDE PLANK

10 to 20 repetitions
page 57

3. STANDING MARCH TO CRUNCH

20 to 30 repetitions
page 77

4. CLIMBING PLANK

8 to 12 repetitions
page 47

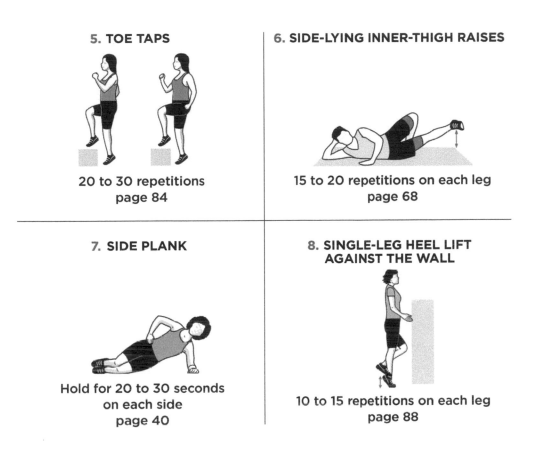

5. TOE TAPS

20 to 30 repetitions
page 84

6. SIDE-LYING INNER-THIGH RAISES

15 to 20 repetitions on each leg
page 68

7. SIDE PLANK

Hold for 20 to 30 seconds
on each side
page 40

8. SINGLE-LEG HEEL LIFT AGAINST THE WALL

10 to 15 repetitions on each leg
page 88

MODIFICATIONS If breathing is a challenge, it can take away from good form; this is especially true for exercises that use multiple body parts. Work at a pace at which you can still hold a conversation, even if it's a breathless one. If you find you can't talk at all during the workout, try doing the lower end of repetitions suggested and rest for 1½ to 2 minutes between each exercise.

TO YOUR LEVEL

If you're mastering this expert program and want to add a metabolic challenge, add a second set of **Standing March to Crunch** and **Toe Taps** at the end of your second circuit to keep your heart rate up.

At the end of your entire workout, test your core strength by seeing how long you can hold a **Low Plank** with good form. Time yourself and write it down. You can try it again in the future to see how your core endurance has improved.

Self Check-In

1. **Is it time for a new pair of sneakers?**
   » *Check out the wear and tear on your workout shoes. If you are wearing them a lot, especially outside your workouts, you might need a new pair in a shorter period than you'd expect—sometimes in as little as four months. Look at it as an investment in your fitness.*

2. **Am I getting enough energy and nutrition from the food I'm eating?**
   » *If you are eating generally healthy food but still don't feel your best, it might be time to add some nutritional supplements. Refer to chapter 2 for more on supplements.*

3. **Am I staying in good form during my workouts?**
   » *If you are unsure, record yourself and take a look. You can also do your workouts in front of a mirror. It's okay to check yourself out!*

4. **Am I getting enough sleep?**
   » *Muscles rebuild and get stronger while you're resting. Recovery is essential to reaching your fitness goals.*

WEEK TWO
expert

Prepare yourself for a greater challenge in this week's workout, as the exercises offered here all require total body strength. Plan for two rest days between these workouts, instead of one. On your rest days, implement some light cardio to keep blood pumping throughout the body and help your muscles recover with movement. Motion is lotion!

Getting a little bit uncomfortable
in your workouts will make
your body more comfortable
for the rest of the day.

Days of the Week: 3 times a week, with two days between workouts

Approximate Time: 30 to 35 minutes, with 5-minute warm-up and 5-minute cooldown

Overview: Complete exercises 1 through 4 to complete one circuit and then repeat for a second circuit. Rest no more than 3 minutes between each circuit. Then complete exercises 5 through 8 for one circuit and then repeat for a second circuit. Rest for 30 to 60 seconds between each exercise.

Warm-Up: Moderate-intensity movement to elevate your core temperature, such as brisk walking, light jogging, aerobics, stairs, or cycling. If time allows, spend an additional 5 minutes increasing your intensity to a more vigorous level.

Cooldown: 4 to 5 upper- and lower-body stretches

1. ECCENTRIC PUSH-UP TO COBRA

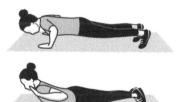

8 to 12 repetitions
page 58

2. BULGARIAN LUNGE

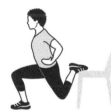

15 to 20 repetitions on each leg
page 83

3. LAT SLIDES

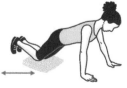

5 to 10 repetitions
page 62

4. PLIE SQUAT

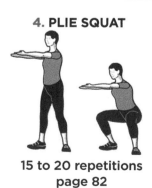

15 to 20 repetitions
page 82

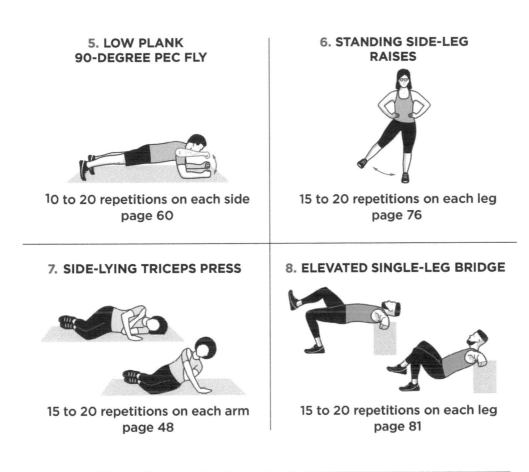

5. LOW PLANK 90-DEGREE PEC FLY

10 to 20 repetitions on each side
page 60

6. STANDING SIDE-LEG RAISES

15 to 20 repetitions on each leg
page 76

7. SIDE-LYING TRICEPS PRESS

15 to 20 repetitions on each arm
page 48

8. ELEVATED SINGLE-LEG BRIDGE

15 to 20 repetitions on each leg
page 81

MODIFICATIONS If you have a history of shoulder injury, consider going only as deep as your elbows on the **Eccentric Push-Up to Cobra** exercise, and then setting up separately to do each Cobra so you don't put undue stress on your shoulder joint.

If you feel knee strain during the **Bulgarian Lunge**, try doing the **Standing Quadriceps Stretch** (page 31) and holding it for 60 seconds before doing this exercise, and limit yourself to a comfortable range of motion.

TO YOUR LEVEL

This circuit starts with an **Eccentric Push-Up to Cobra**, which emphasizes a slowing of movement when you are going in the same direction as gravity. For a greater challenge to the entire circuit, try slowing down the eccentric phase during every exercise, not just that first one. This means you'll want to move very slowly when gravity is on your side and forcefully push when working against gravity. Try counting to 4 on the way down and 1 on the way up.

Self Check-In

1. **Am I eating five or more fruits and vegetables a day?**
   » *It's recommended by the USDA to eat five to nine servings of fruits and vegetables a day.*

2. **Have I been steadily increasing the number of sets and reps completed?**
   » *You don't have to go to complete muscle exertion to see results, but it's best to occasionally work past your perceived limits. Think of it this way: It's impossible to do more every time, but try to do more sometimes.*

3. **Do I have a daily routine that includes my workout?**
   » *Motivation comes and goes for all of us, but discipline will keep you in the game. Make exercise part of a daily routine that you insist upon.*

4. **Am I getting enough movement on non-workout days?**
   » *In addition to your workouts, try to get an additional hour of walking. This can be accumulated throughout the day, so maybe take a ten-minute walking break every hour for six hours if you're sitting most of the day.*

WEEK THREE
expert

This is your final week of expert programs. This double-circuit workout is a lot of fun. The leg exercises work out your whole body and will keep your heart rate up and challenge your balance. The core and arm exercises will demonstrate how far you've come with arm strength, abdominal endurance, and shoulder stability. Even though you're an expert, listen to your body. No matter how fit you are, it's possible to encounter areas of weakness and imbalance. When this happens, it's absolutely fine (and recommended) to slow things down, take a step back, and take care of yourself.

Be proud of yourself.
You've come a long way
and have created a lifestyle
that will serve you well.

Days of the Week: 3 times a week, with two days between workouts

Approximate Time: 30 to 35 minutes, with 5-minute warm-up and 5-minute cooldown

Overview: Complete exercises 1 through 4 to complete one circuit and then repeat for a second circuit. Rest no more than 3 minutes between each circuit. Then complete exercises 5 through 8 for one circuit and then repeat for a second circuit. Rest for 30 to 60 seconds between each exercise.

Warm-Up: Moderate-intensity movement to elevate your core temperature, such as brisk walking, light jogging, aerobics, stairs, or cycling. If time allows, spend an additional 5 minutes increasing your intensity to a more vigorous level.

Cooldown: 4 to 5 upper- and lower-body stretches

1. LATERAL BOUNDS

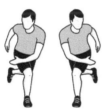

20 to 30 repetitions
page 72

2. INVERTED SCAPULA PRESS-UP

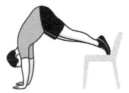

10 to 15 repetitions
page 52

3. BULGARIAN LUNGE

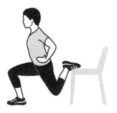

15 to 20 repetitions on each leg
page 83

4. TRICEPS DIP STRAIGHT LEG

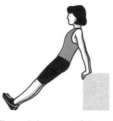

15 to 20 repetitions
page 46

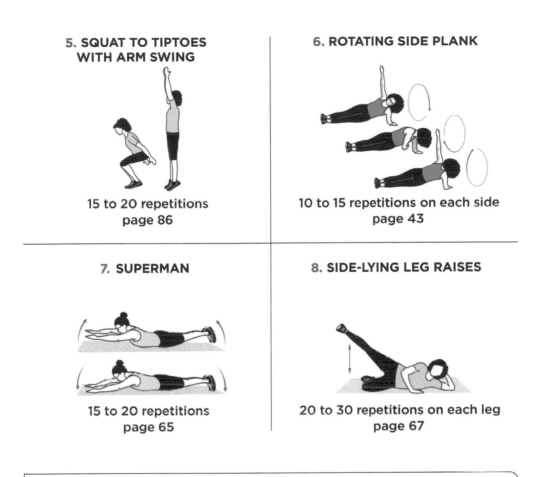

**5. SQUAT TO TIPTOES
WITH ARM SWING**

15 to 20 repetitions
page 86

6. ROTATING SIDE PLANK

10 to 15 repetitions on each side
page 43

7. SUPERMAN

15 to 20 repetitions
page 65

8. SIDE-LYING LEG RAISES

20 to 30 repetitions on each leg
page 67

MODIFICATIONS At this point in your workout progressions, expect your form to be solid for every exercise in this circuit. If you feel shaky, slow things down and stick with the lower end of suggested repetitions—this is still beneficial. Look back over the details in chapter 3 to make sure you're doing the exercises properly. Even experts can always benefit from checking their foundation for cracks.

TO YOUR LEVEL

For a greater challenge on these circuits, try to cut your rest time to 30 seconds between exercises and 60 seconds between circuits. Maintain a reasonable speed on the exercises themselves because you don't want to lose form or the time your muscles need under tension for development.

Self Check-In

1.   **Do I have all proper tools in place to keep exercise in my life for good?**

    » *You don't need much, but it can help to have a good exercise mat, decent exercise shoes, a robust support system, and a generally positive attitude.*

2.   **Do I feel worn out or fatigued?**

    » *Just because you're strong enough to do a hard workout doesn't mean every workout has to be hard. It's okay to go back to basics or take it easy for a week and do some less strenuous movement. Listen to your body.*

3.   **How are my health stats?**

    » *When was your last physical? It's a good idea to see a doctor annually to make sure you're doing everything you can to take care of your health and there are no underlying issues. And after twelve weeks of regular work-outs, a visit to the doc will show the positive effects of exercise on your vital signs.*

4.   **Am I getting enough good nutrition, hydration, sleep, and movement?**

    » *These are the key components to staying fit and healthy. Seek a balance of all four of these things.*

Expert Program Notes

Use these pages to take down notes for each week of your workout. Reflect on your strengths and weaknesses. Do you have favorite exercises? Exercises that need some extra work? Did you notice any trends on days you felt particularly good? Did certain meals affect your workouts?

WEEK ONE

WEEK TWO

WEEK THREE

STRENGTH AS A PRACTICE, NOT AS A GOAL

An exercise is just an exercise, but in this chapter, we'll lay the groundwork for you to keep bodyweight training in your life forever as a *lifestyle*. You'll find suggestions for how to build your own workout once you have completed all the workouts in this book. We'll also go over some things to look out for and discuss self-monitoring as it applies to your future workouts. Following this is a list of resources to further support you on your lifelong journey with fitness and good health.

WHAT'S NEXT?

You've stayed the course and put yourself through twelve weeks of bodyweight training. It's a major accomplishment, and the best way to reward yourself is to keep going. Let this be the beginning of a lifelong love affair with your fitness routine. Over time, the more you give to it, the more you'll receive in a myriad of lifelong benefits.

Take a moment to back to chapter 4 and revisit some of the first workouts you did. You'll remember those first few weeks and discover how much stronger your foundation is now and how much easier it is to get through the basics. Repeat your favorite workouts as often as you like, and keep yourself challenged by adding a few extra reps or a whole extra set. You can also pick some of your favorite exercises and create your own circuit. Just try to create total-body workouts to keep things in balance.

On some days, let yourself have fun and enjoy getting some muscle-stimulating movement. Not every workout needs to take you to the next level. Just remember that leaving your comfort zone and working out at least twice a week with regularity will deliver the greatest benefits.

Self-Study for a Strong Life

Regular self-reflection on your health and fitness can be preventive as well. For example, take ongoing notes on your exercise life. This can keep you motivated; it can also help you identify areas of weakness that could lead to injury. Muscle fatigue is expected at times, but joint pain or radiating nerve pain is not. If something aches and then worsens with exercise, contact a doctor, and in the meantime, avoid the exercises that exacerbate the pain until you have a treatment plan. Get regular check-ups and always listen to your body. Modern activity trackers monitor your heart rate and other vital signs and can alert you to issues that require medical treatment. Dizziness, inability to catch your breath, and chest pain while you are working out are always reasons to contact a doctor immediately. As we've explored, lots of things impact physical fitness: stress, sleep, nutrition, hydration, and of course, exercise. Keep these aspects of health in mind and consider how you can improve each one.

Build Your Community

Beyond the workouts in this book, or any workouts, it's important to keep an overall active lifestyle for general wellness and vitality. Many people find it easier to stay fit and active when surrounded by others who share the same goal. Find people who will help you stay more active. Invite your friends to join you for a walk or hike instead of meeting for coffee at the diner. Maybe there is someone you can join a yoga studio with or partner up with in a social sport like tennis. Participate in community fitness events, like 5Ks for charity. You'll be giving back to your community and yourself at the same time. As you intentionally put yourself in more active situations, you'll meet people of all ages who are prioritizing their health and enjoying the journey. Having active, healthy friends helps you stay active.

Listen to Your Body

Just because you have expertly done all the workouts in this book doesn't mean that you have to do the hardest moves at your highest level all the time. Bodyweight exercise training is a practice for you to have for life; you won't be continuously growing and leveling up on a weekly basis. Sometimes your body needs a rest, and sometimes your foundation needs some maintenance. You can still stay active and challenge yourself in different ways. Try to set the hardest programs aside for a month, and come back to them after engaging in some more basic programs or focusing on another aspect of your fitness like flexibility, stretches, or cardiovascular strength. You might find that when you return to your expert programs, you have broken through to a new high you didn't expect.

Enjoy All That Strength Has to Offer

I am so proud of you for picking up this book and choosing a stronger, healthier life. Thank you for joining me and keep up the terrific work. I know it isn't easy to start something new or even to find room in your life to prioritize yourself. When you take care of yourself, you are taking care of others. You are making yourself a stronger, healthier, and more energetic person. You'll have more of yourself to give to the people in your life you care about the most. On some days, it might seem impossible to find thirty minutes to dedicate to yourself, but remember that it's buying you time later. Your workouts are a long-term investment in your health and well-being. Please have patience—it may take time to see rewards, but they will come. And as you grow more confident in your fitness, you'll find you're gaining freedom in mobility, which will help you maintain your independence as you age. In the meantime, I think you're awesome.

CLOSING
Stay Strong

I hope you've had fun with the workouts in this book, and I hope you'll keep it as a reference. Don't keep your fitness a secret—share it and get others to join you. Who knows? Maybe now *you're* the fitness role model to whom everyone is coming to for advice.

The quest for health and happiness is a lifelong endeavor, and, because life happens, unexpected challenges will come up along the way. Stay committed to maintaining your strength in changing situations, because no matter your age, every pitfall you may encounter will be easier to overcome in a strong body. Keep finding ways to have fun, and be your own biggest supporter. Your body is a powerful and magical thing—nurture it and treat it with compassion and care. With your positive mindset, consistency, and determination, you can do anything.

GLOSSARY

(bodyweight) circuit training: A workout combination in which different exercises are done back-to-back with short rest periods between them to make up a total body routine

calcium: A mineral your body needs to maintain strong bones; helps carry out other important cellular functions

carbohydrates: One of the three main nutrients found in food; they break down to glucose in the body, becoming your body's main source of energy

cardiovascular: Relating to the heart and blood vessels

cardiovascular training: Exercise focused on improving heart health and endurance by increasing core temperature and heart rate

collagen: The main structural protein found in skin and connective body tissues

diabetes: A disease that causes the body to have abnormal production of and responses to the hormone insulin

glucose: A simple sugar and component of many carbohydrates; also an important energy source

hypertension: High blood pressure

lean body mass: Total bodyweight that is not body fat

macronutrients: The three essential nutrients needed for body function: carbohydrates, fat, and protein

magnesium: A mineral your body needs to maintain normal cell function, support healthy immune system function, and keep bones strong

micronutrients: Nutrients that your body needs in smaller amounts; usually referred to as vitamins and minerals

myofascial release: A manual therapy technique aimed at releasing tension in muscular connective tissue

neurological: Relating to the nerves or nervous system of the body

osteoarthritis: A disease characterized by joint degeneration in which the cartilage and underlying bone break down, leading to pain and stiffness

osteoporosis: A medical condition characterized by low bone density, which causes bones to become weak and brittle

perimenopause: The period of a woman's life leading up to menopause when the ovaries start to produce less estrogen, causing various hormonal symptoms

peripheral heart action training: A type of resistance training with cardiovascular benefits; achieved by alternating between upper- and lower-body exercises

protein: A nutrient made up of many amino acids, found in food like meat, eggs, and beans. It is an essential part of the diet for normal cell function.

resistance training: A strength-training program where external resistance (such as that provided by dumbbells, resistance bands, medicine balls, etc.) is added to movement to stimulate muscle growth

sarcopenia: A reduction in muscle mass due to aging

static stretches: Stretches in which you hold a single stretched position for 30 to 60 seconds

weight training: Lifting weights in a training program to improve strength and muscle mass

ONLINE

ACE: Free Exercise Library and Resources

ACEFitness.org

The American Council on Exercise is the industry standard for personal trainers and group exercise instructors. This website contains a free exercise library with detailed descriptions and photographs of hundreds of exercises. It'll also connect you with ACE experts all around the United States.

AllTrails

Explore hiking trails near and far. The free version of this app lets you explore and discover your local hiking adventures with detailed descriptions of intensity and accessibility.

Calm

An app to help with sleep quality, relaxation, and meditation. Free trial and annual membership.

Do Yoga with Me

DoYogaWithMe.com

Expert yoga instructional videos for all levels. Both free online material and subscription-based classes.

***Fat-Burning Man* Podcast**

Fitness and nutrition expert Abel James interviews industry leaders, health gurus, and doctors about health.

Headspace

An app to help with sleep quality, relaxation, and meditation. Free trial and monthly subscription.

Lose It!

Excellent weight-loss app and calorie tracker.

Nutrition.gov
The USDA-sponsored website for nutrition, offering the latest information to help you make healthy food choices.

Runkeeper
Want to start running or take your step counting to a higher level? This app helps you understand mileage and pacing, record your workouts, and join an online running community.

Web MD: Myofascial Release Therapy Resource
WebMD.com/pain-management/what-to-know-myofascial-release-therapy

This website explains myofascial tissue, benefits of this massage, and self-massage techniques.

Yoga with Adriene
YogaWithAdriene.com

Connect to curated yoga playlists on Adriene's YouTube channel to find the right free yoga workouts for you.

BOOKS

***Fitness Over 40: A 6-Week Exercise Plan to Build Endurance, Strength, and Flexibility* by Stefanie Lisa**
This book provides a simple and balanced exercise program that preserves energy, builds strength, and prevents age-related frailty.

***Strength Training Over 40: A 6-Week Program to Build Muscle and Agility* by Alana Collins**
This book offers a structured program for building total body strength using both gym and home equipment.

REFERENCES

Cotton, Richard T., and Ross E. Anderson. *Clinical Exercise Specialist Manual.* San Diego: American Council on Exercise, 1999.

Godman, Heidi. "Regular Exercise Changes the Brain to Improve Memory, Thinking Skills." Harvard Health, April 9, 2014. health.harvard.edu/blog /regular-exercise-changes-brain-improve-memory-thinking-skills -201404097110.

Hayes, Kim. "How Much Protein Do You Need After 50?" AARP Healthy Living, February 12, 2018. aarp.org/health/healthy-living/info-2018/protein -needs-fd.

Hörder, H. et al. "Midlife Cardiovascular Fitness and Dementia: A 44-Year Longitudinal Population Study in Women." *Neurology* 90, no. 15 (April 10, 2018): e1298–e1305. ePub March 14, 2018, PubMed. alzforum.org/news /research-news/44-year-study-ties-midlife-fitness-lower-dementia-risk.

Landsverk, Gary. "Doing Too Many HIIT Workouts a Week Can Hurt Your Metabolism and Destabilize Your Blood Sugar, a Small Study Suggests." Insider.com, May 24, 2021. insider.com/overdoing-hiit-workouts-metabolism -backfire-fitness-study-suggests-2021-3.

Pratesi, Alessandra, Francesca Tarantini, and Mauro Di Bari. "Skeletal Muscle: An Endocrine Organ." CCMBM, May 2013, US National Library of Medicine. doi.org/10.11138/ccmbm/2013.10.1.011.

Samuels, Vickie. *Foundation in Kinesiology and Biomechanics*, Philadelphia: F. A. Davis Company, 2018.

INDEX

ACKNOWLEDGMENTS

Thanks to my always loving and endlessly supportive family, especially Dan and Emily, for letting me take the time to write this book. Also, thanks to my clients and friends who give me inspiration daily to keep exercise fresh, creative, and important in my own life so I can share it with them.

ABOUT THE AUTHOR

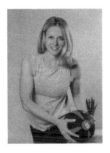 **MEL McGUIRE** is a personal trainer, group fitness instructor, and founder of Joyful Fitness CT (JoyfulFitnessCT.com). She has eighteen years of experience working with clients of all ages and fitness levels. She is certified as a personal trainer by the National Strength & Conditioning Association and the National Academy of Sports Medicine. She is a certified Medical Exercise Specialist through the American Council on Exercise. She also holds a bachelor's degree in music from New York University. Mel lives in Stamford, Connecticut, with her husband, stepdaughter, son, and three fur babies. Connect with her on Instagram @joyfulfitness.